GET ON TOP

OF YOUR PLEASURE, SEXUALITY & WELLNESS

A Vagina Revolution

....

MEIKA HOLLENDER

with Alexandra Zissu

TOUCHSTONE

New York London Toronto Sydney New Delhi

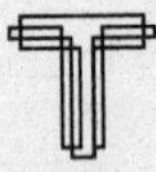

Touchstone
An Imprint of Simon & Schuster, Inc.
1230 Avenue of the Americas
New York, NY 10020

First Touchstone trade paperback edition March 2018

TOUCHSTONE and colophon are trademarks of Simon & Schuster, Inc.

For information about special discounts for bulk purchases, please contact Simon & Schuster Special Sales at 1-866-506-1949 or business@simonandschuster.com.

The Simon & Schuster Speakers Bureau can bring authors to your live event. For more information or to book an event, contact the Simon & Schuster Speakers Bureau at 1-212-698-8888 or visit our website at www.SimonSpeakers.com.

Interior design by Jaime Putorti

Manufactured in the United States of America

10 9 8 7 6 5 4 3 2 1

Library of Congress Cataloging-in-Publication Data is available.

ISBN 978-1-5011-7997-6
ISBN 978-1-5011-7998-3 (ebook)

Advance praise for
Meika Hollender and *Get on Top*

"Imagine your high school sex ed class (if you even had one) flipped on its head. We can't get enough of the sex-positive, normalizing way Meika writes about sex and sexual health and shares relevant information that you can actually use."

—Laura McQuade, President and CEO,
Planned Parenthood of New York City

"Meika Hollender is making sex healthier for everyone."

—Girlboss.com

"Meika Hollender has a way of turning topics that make some blush into conversations that we can all join. Only a woman that has the foresight to build Sustain and the 'Get On Top' national campaign would have the insight to write this book. From one #Girlboss to a world of #Girlbosses, *Get on Top* answers REAL questions, is accessible, informative, smart, and necessary."

—Skylar Diggins-Smith, WNBA All-Star

"Meika Hollender has taken everything she has learned building Sustain and created sex ed for the #Girlboss generation. Meika is the ultimate #Girlboss who empowers us all with her rally cry to "Get On Top." I'm buying one for every woman (and girlboss in the making) I know!"

—Christy Turlington Burns, Founder
and CEO, Every Mother Counts

"Meika Hollender's *Get on Top* is not only a guide to sexual health for millennials but a call to action for all women to take control of their bodies."

—Jeanne Rizzo, RN, President and CEO,
Breast Cancer Prevention Partners

"Meika has written an invaluable resource for women in an age of misinformation and uncertainty. As founder of Sustain Natural, she's sparked a candid dialogue around safe and all-natural sexual wellness, and *Get on Top* furthers this important mission to destigmatize sexual health."

—Katherine Ryder, Founder and CEO, Maven

"With #GetOnTop, Sustain's founder, Meika Hollender, is aiming to squash the stigma surrounding women and sexual health, and elevate a national conversation to encourage women to take control of their sexual experience."

—*Women's Health*

CONTENTS

GET ON TOP

INTRODUCTION

My name is Meika, and I'm on a mission to destigmatize female sexuality. Entirely. To connect women to their sexual health and help them care for and get to know their bodies. To hold them up. To normalize what should already be normal.

The primary way I'm doing this is through Sustain, a sexual-wellness company I founded with my dad, because who didn't grow up dreaming of selling condoms with their father? OK, not me, but I do just that.

I know. It's a jarring bit of information, or so people tell me. It begs context, so let's back it up.

A few years ago, when I was finishing business school at NYU Stern, my dad approached me with an idea he had many years ago. He wanted to start a sustainable condom company. I know most people find a family condom company kind of weird, but stay with me here. My family has deep, deep roots in the sustainable products world. More than thirty years ago my parents founded Seventh Generation. We also have a long-standing commitment to women's health. When Seventh Generation introduced organic cotton tampons, I—then a teenager—was super involved. By that I mean I, among other things, drove around in the Seventh Generation "tamponification" mobile for an entire summer (think green tampon fairies painted on a white Prius). I got passionate about reproductive health and involved with Planned Parenthood at a very young age. Women's sexual health became part of my DNA. Now more than ever I feel like we all need to be talking about it. All day, every day. We're under siege.

I'll spare you the business details, but I do want to explain why condoms were of particular interest. Oddly, the manufacture of and ingredients used in sexual-wellness products, including condoms and lubricant (Sustain makes that, too, plus organic cotton tampons, pads, and personal care products), can harm rather than help bodies. There are potentially harmful chemicals and residues in the resulting products, which is of particular concern considering these intimate products are going inside our bodies. So my father and I saw an important opportunity to create better, safer, healthier products. Then I decided to follow my passion and focus on women, like no other condom brand has done ever.

I arrived at clarity around this mission for our business over time. It went something like this. First off, when I approached the condom market from a female perspective, in our earliest days of founding the company, I learned some pretty terrifying statistics.

Did you know:

- Only 21 percent of single women use condoms regularly.
- 48 percent of pregnancies are unplanned.
- One in four college freshmen contract an STI.*

I also learned that 70 percent of women feel uncomfortable buying condoms, which is pretty wild because 40 percent of condoms are actually purchased by women.

Have you ever been in a condom aisle? It for sure feels anything but vagina-friendly. I felt fire-under-my-feet compelled to fix that. I can't even explain how incredibly important it has been to create a brand and a movement that empowers women to feel proud of their sexuality and to get on top of their sexual health, with no stigma attached.

The initial reaction to Sustain was thrilling: retailers responded to the first brand of female-focused, natural sexual-

---

* All facts and figures in the following pages come from the kickass resources listed on pages 235–236.

wellness products by saying it was addressing a hole in the market. We were filling a need!

Right around then something crappy happened, and it was the best type of gut check. Just before Sustain officially launched, in 2014, we landed a piece of press on a major media website. The minute I got the link from our PR agency, I clicked through to the article, and excitement flooded over me. That was a super brief moment because then I scrolled down to the bottom of the article, and started reading through the comments.

You can't see me right now, but I have a not-small freckle on my lower lip. The first comment was: "What's that on her lip? Is that an STD? Clearly she should be using condoms, not selling them!"

Verbatim.

And you know what? This painful/idiotic response and the sexism inherent in it were not isolated. There was that time on a plane when the guy next to me mistook what I did as selling real estate because he just couldn't believe a young woman would sell what I sell. I had to inform him that, sir, sorry, I sell condoms not condos. I can't believe people are still so awkward about sex. Our culture is overtly sexual while also sexually repressed in so many ways. I guess it shouldn't be a surprise. We've been repressing women for centuries in every country around the world. So many women don't even know what their own vaginas look like, or how best to take care of them. Sex, even safe sex, is a taboo subject. All of these experiences have strengthened my resolve and boosted my drive to do my work.

I'm here to shift the dynamics. I want women to be familiar with their own bodies, and to make sex un-taboo, especially as, due to a combo of not enough and horribly laughable sex education in America, rising rates of STIs, including HIV (particularly among young people), and the patriarchy, our country appears to need a major wake-up call when it comes to women's health. The more I travel and talk to people about Sustain, the clearer it becomes: our society—even today—still labels a girl who carries a condom a slut and a guy who does the same a hero.

Add that to the lists of things I will change.

What I can't change—though give me time—is the sexual education you had before you picked up this book. If you can't remember a single thing you'd be able to technically call sex ed, beyond a lackluster period talk with a gym teacher and maybe a few confusing nights groping with a first boyfriend or girlfriend, you're not alone. Sexual education is not mandatory in the United States. There is no standardized curriculum, like there is in other enlightened countries, including the Netherlands. (They start in kindergarten!) In 2016, only twenty-two states and the District of Columbia mandated both sex and HIV education, two states mandated sex education alone, and another twelve states mandated only HIV education. While thirty-seven states specifically require that sex education include abstinence, a sum total of zero states require that contraception be the focus, and only thirteen states require that the information being taught is *medically accurate*. How scary is that? And yet of course all the public health and various medical professional organizations that count (you know, American Medical Association, American Academy of Pediatrics, etc.) support a comprehensive approach to sex ed. Without science and a standardized curriculum, a lot of room is left for the personal opinion of whatever adult is tasked with "instructing" impressionable young people about reproduction, bodily changes, periods, and sex. Unfortunately that includes unfounded information, especially about sex—freaky guilt-inducing psychology and just plain wrong details. Maybe you were told something by a friend's older sibling, or your parents ponied up some watered-down nuggets of information. Maybe whatever you know about sex came from your oversharing hot-to-trot aunt, or from a buttoned-up church elder. Chances are there was a big, strong emphasis on not getting pregnant and very little on hormones or anatomy, including vocabulary. And for sure no one ever mentioned pleasure. Probably sex mainly sounded transactional, something along the lines of *A penis goes in a vagina and the girl gets pregnant. The end.* Presumably no one suggested you sit yourself down in front of a mirror and give yourself a good long look or talked about vaginal health or masturbation or lust or love or friendship or the differences and similarities between men and women's desire or that it's perfectly normal—and even a good idea—to talk about sex. Often and openly.

You can change all that today, by choosing to make pleasure a focus and by getting to know your body. Though it's also important to understand that this can be easier said than done. When generations of young people stumble into their sexual lives with very little information and are too embarrassed to talk about sex but have 24/7 access to the Internet, weird things happen. Like porn obsession, rampant STIs, and slut shaming. These are real problems, even though right at this very moment there's a fantastic growing cultural movement of sex positivity, of being anti–slut shaming. We're kind of a mess about sex. Like, there's Gwyneth Paltrow's team writing about the joys of lube and anal on her website, Goop, but some actresses are still running around like old-school pinup girls, their worth in the world mainly related to how sexy they appear. And then there's our government trying to defund Planned Parenthood. We have a vice president, at the time of this writing, who won't eat alone with any women other than his wife, and a president who feels it's OK to grab women by their pussies. The #MeToo movement is rapidly ferreting out and taking down sexual harassers in every industry from Hollywood to journalism and beyond. There are endless date-rape cases rocking college campuses across the country, thrusting the critical issue of consent onto the front pages of newspapers, websites, and magazines everywhere. And on campuses like Yale, where the students are ostensibly smart, there are fraternities suspended for years on end after the "brothers" were found chanting active calls for sexual assault: *No means yes! Yes means anal!* To add to this fractured collective sexuality, there's Tinder—people can easily swipe right to sex at any moment of the day, with any number of partners, plus lots and lots of dick pics. So despite progress happening on many fronts, we somehow, as a country, still aren't fundamentally comfortable about sex and sexuality—especially women's sexuality.

Here's what is clear: women are sexual beings and should feel free to embrace this. In fact, the clitoris is the only body part—male or female—whose only purpose is pleasure. It has more sensory nerve endings than the penis. Also? It's similar in size to a penis. It goes way beyond the hooded nub most people refer to as a clit (more on that on page 17). But we have our own kind of sexuality. Imagine if there were standardized sex ed *and* it included information about how and why sex feels good. And girls and boys learned—starting young—not just about pregnancy and disease but also about masturbation and orgasm and that regular old penis-in-vagina sex results in orgasm for only 30 percent of women because of *anatomy*. And that for the remaining 70 percent there are a lot of fun (and safe) other ways to play.

This is science. This is black-and-white fact. What if the mark of losing your virginity was when you had your first orgasm with a partner—not penetration? What if we let young adults know that emotions and being comfortable with a partner play a big role in sexuality and pleasure? The brain is really the root of sexuality when it comes down to it—the center of desire. One study showed that 38 percent of college-aged women don't enjoy first sexual encounters (hi, Tinder), but by six months with the same partner, 68 percent of these women are enjoying themselves.

With better information, and a level of comfort that comes with communication, that number can be higher. And it can be achieved with women's health in mind. Sex and wellness should go hand in hand. Sex is good for you—especially when practiced safely. I can't tell you how badly I want women not only to buy, carry, and use condoms, but also to feel great about doing so. I created a campaign around this very topic and launched it during Women's Health Week 2016 (#GetOnTop). I felt a personal responsibility to create a way to enable women to talk about sex and feel comfortable doing it. So I got together nine female founders—ranging from an eco-activist to the cofounder of *Refinery29*—to film a short video about sex and sexual health. My goal was to get one hundred thousand women to pledge to practice safe sex.

Within hours of launching the campaign, thousands of women from all over the world were pledging to "get on top" of their health and practice safe sex. I was interviewed by everyone from Fox News to *Fast Company* and people just seemed to get it. Did we reach one hundred thousand pledges right away? Not quite. But people are talking. If Sustain shut down tomorrow, I know I will at least have started a vitally important conversation. Keeping this conversation going is everything.

Sustain, thankfully, is very much alive. And I have tons of work to do. A few months after we launched the pledge, I got invited to do a Tumblr "Answer Time," fielding questions from women about all things sexual health. I thought it would be a breeze. I mean, at that point I had probably answered five thousand sex-related questions in real time. But then the queries started rolling in. And I was struck. I was so taken off guard. Because you know what? Women are suffering. Women, especially in the eighteen-to-thirty age range—but older and younger, too—are suffering from misinformation, fear, intimidation. They're suffering from vaginal dryness, or are too anxious to talk to their partners, or can't understand why sex hurts. They're worried about side effects of birth control, confused by pimples on their vulvas, don't know what—if any—soap to use to wash themselves, don't know when or always even where to seek medical attention. They're confused about consent, sexuality, odors, cheating. They want answers about chlamydia, masturbation, pregnancy scares, and what it means to be a slut. They really want to know why if they can orgasm with a vibrator, how come it's not also happening with oral or penetration. They really, really need answers from someone they trust. From a partner.

I want to be that partner. I want to help women get cliterate. I want to help them access all the facts they need to make smart, healthy, and safe choices when it comes to sex, and I don't mean by selling them organic lubricant (though everyone should have some—lube is for sure the short answer to most of those pain questions!). I mean by continuing the conversation, by helping them tune in and think with their vaginas, by answering questions, by providing the information I have access to in a relatable and totally normal way. Not sexed up, not sleazy, not patronizing, not dumbed down. Just smart, actionable information for any and all vagina-related questions. Not clinical, but rooted in science. Un-self-conscious, straightforward, real, and enlightening. And all of this information delivered in a pro-pleasure, safety-first, and empowering sex-positive way.

And that's exactly what the following pages are all about.

Meika Hollender

CHAPTER 1

FIRST THINGS FIRST: GETTING TO KNOW YOUR VAGINA

Your vagina is a wonderland. It's time to learn exactly what that means. It's crazy how few of us know our own ins and outs and how many times you hear anecdotes that even grown women don't know they have three holes, not two. No, we don't pee out of our vaginas. If you want to get technical, it isn't your vagina at all. It's your vulva. The vagina is literally the curved canal that various things can go into and out of, if you so desire (e.g., fingers, penises, toys, tampons, speculums, babies, etc.). But since many people don't even know what their parts are called, let alone what they look like, we all just call our vulvas vaginas. And so we're stuck with grouping all our complex and wonderful genital parts into one: *vagina*. You can, of course, call them whatever you want. They're yours. The better you know you, the better you can love your parts for all they are. If you're intimately aware of what your vagina, vulva, and clitoris are like when they're healthy—how they operate, smell, feel, function—you'll more easily be able to identify if and when something is off.

By the way, it's important to note that female equipment is incredible. Amazing. What men have doesn't even come close, not that this is a competition. It's just that the female reproductive system and sexual organs are basically superheroes, something to be in awe of. Almost all women have the same parts, but they're all configured a little differently. Like, here's one example, but yours might look a little or a lot different. If you're game, take a moment to check out your vagina and all of its surrounding marvels. Grab a mirror and go for it.

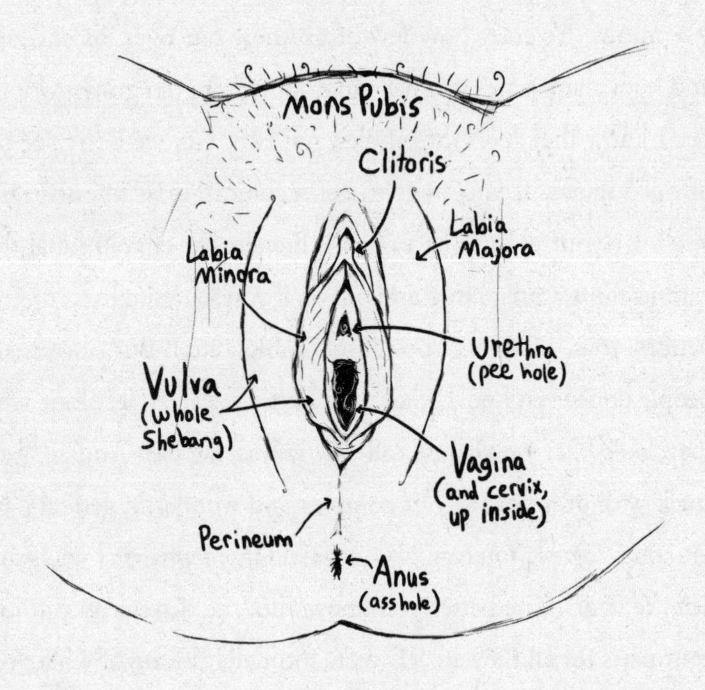

VULVA: This is the whole external shebang—from lips to clit, it's all vulva.

MONS PUBIS: That's the puffy part where the pubes are, just above your pubic bone. Some people have more meat here than others.

LABIA MAJORA: These are the exterior lips—the fleshier ones covered in hair. The skin on these is like the skin on the rest of our bodies.

LABIA MINORA: These are your interior lips—the thinner ones with no hair and made from mucous membrane. The skin on these is more like the skin in our mouths. Some people have longer ones than others. On some women, you can see these inner lips kind of protruding from the outer lips. On other women, you have to spread the majora to see the minora. They come in many colors, shapes, and sizes. One lip may even be longer than the other. They have a protective role: keeping bacteria and the like out of other connecting parts. And they have a sexual role: filled with nerve endings and quite sensitive, these inner lips can be critical to arousal.

CLITORIS: To check out this goddess and get fully cliterate, spread your labia and peek below the mons pubis. There you will see your clitoral hood. Under that is a nub of the clit called the glans. Most people think that's it, but this is just the tip of the iceberg (literally). Your actual clitoris goes much farther back than that nub internally, running basically like two legs (called crura) under the labia majora. It kind of looks like a wishbone, with the ends of the legs hanging over something called the vestibular bulbs. These are also internal—they surround the vaginal opening beneath the inner labia. Guess what? They're made of erectile tissue, like penises. So when you're having vaginal sex, these bulbs and the crura are what trigger clitoral stimulation. The clit—glans, crura, and vestibular bulbs—is, amazingly, the only organ, male or female, designed solely for sexual pleasure.

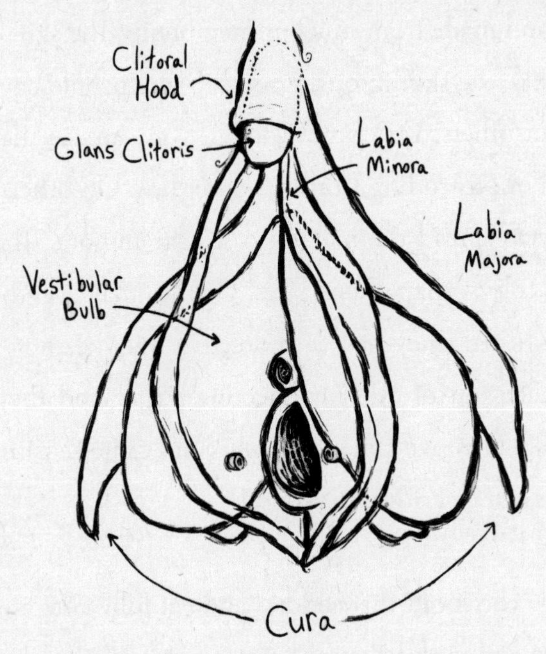

URETHRA: That's the small hole the pee comes out of. If you're someone who "squirts" when you orgasm (see page 205), this is where fluid (it's not pee) is expelled.

VAGINA: Check out the gateway to your vagina. It's a super stretchy spot, so even though it's big enough to pass a baby, you won't be looking at an open hole. Its resting state is closed. Even when you wear tampons, have vaginal sex, or both, it can sometimes be covered partially with some hymen (basically, skin that covers the vaginal canal) or there could be a circle just around the opening that is hymen. If you've had children, you won't likely see hymen tissue any longer. When you have your period, this is where it comes out. The actual vagina is internal—inside the opening. It's strong and flexible. The groups of muscles that surround it are capable of holding tampons in place and squeezing to stop the flow of your pee. Basically it's the space between the external parts you can see and the internal parts you can't: the uterus, tubes, and ovaries. Oh, and, it just so happens to house the G-spot. More on that in chapter six.

PERINEUM: The most interesting part of this pelvic tissue where your tailbone and pubic bones basically meet is called the perineal body. You know it as that spot between your vagina and your asshole, commonly referred to as your taint or your tween. It kind of gets dismissed as a no-(wo)man's-land, but actually there's a fair amount of nerve activity that stems from the pudendal nerve here. The length of the taint differs from woman to woman. There's actually a point to this space: it helps protect your vagina from poop entering it.

ASSHOLE: You know what this is, right? The final stop on the gastrointestinal tract. It's quite flexible, just like the vagina. Its resting state is similarly closed.

CERVIX: You won't be able to see this on your body, but stick a (clean!) finger or two up your vagina and see if you can feel something deep inside that's kind of like the tip of a nose, but with a dent or a dimple. That's it, the opening to the uterus. This is how sperm seeking to fertilize an egg enter your reproductive system. It's also where your uterine lining comes through monthly during your period, and it's what opens during labor to allow a baby to pass. But it doesn't let stuff enter in the other direction; the cervix blocks anything like a tampon inside the vagina from passing into the uterus.

VAGINAL MAINTENANCE

Now that you're on top of your female anatomy, it's time to talk about how to take good care of what you've got. This is similar to what you want to do for the rest of your body: get lots of sleep, drink copious amounts of water, treat it gently, don't do anything risky or unsafe, and work out regularly. But since we're talking about vaginas here, there tends to be a lot of misinformation on how best to accomplish these tasks. And there's a fair amount of stuff anyone with a vagina is dealing with, like discharge and odor. So here's the skinny on pruning, trimming, cleaning, and all around treating your vagina like the badass body part it is.

NICKNAMES

Pussy	Snatch	Yoni
Down there	Crotch	Cunt
Poon	Down under	Beaver
Vajayjay	Vajeen	Pink taco
Honeypot	Bearded clam	Box
Hoo-ha	Furburger	Lady business

VAGINAS ARE NOT SUPPOSED TO BE DRY

You know you have it. That clear or white gooey stuff in your underwear. It's discharge. Everyone with a vagina has discharge, so it's time we all start talking about it more. Vaginas, like mouths, are wet, and that's a good thing.

Here's the deal with discharge: basically it's the vagina and cervix's way of cleaning themselves. As our trusted adviser, Dr. Angela, ob-gyn, says, a vagina is a self-cleaning oven. Discharge comes from the cervix and is made up of stuff we all have in our bodies: water, mucus, cells, sweat, various secretions. It's also hormonal, which means that, depending on where you are in your cycle, the quality and quantity of your discharge will change. Sometimes it's thinner, sometimes it's thicker, more mucus-like.

Around the time of ovulation, women tend to produce a lot and it looks kind of like egg whites or even, some say, jellyfish. This happens so sperm can more readily move through it, which is great if you're trying to get pregnant. If not, knowing when you're likely most fertile (aka sperm-friendly) just by reading your cervical mucus is a cool trick. Some women create very little discharge; others say they make a large amount. It's all good.

The more familiar you are with your regular discharge, the easier it will be for you to identify when something is off. The only reason you should ever worry about discharge is if you're having itching or burning, it smells bad, it's heavy and chunky, or it's a funky color. For most people, the yellowish dried crust on your undies does not constitute a funky color. That's just what happens to white or clear discharge when the moisture evaporates out. Gray, green, even pinkish with blood spots? That's funky. For that, you need to visit your gynecologist.

Some women find discharge incredibly annoying. They don't like feeling wet all the time, so they wear liners to absorb the moisture. If you choose to do that, avoid liners made with synthetic materials (see page 69) and especially ones with added perfume; these can irritate your sensitive skin. And don't forget to change the liners often. You don't want constant moisture all stuck up there. You could end up with a rash. And sure, discharge can be annoying, but consider that at some point when you age and your estrogen decreases and you go through menopause, it's going to drastically dry up. And, by all reports, you'll miss it. So enjoy it while you've got it.

A WELL-BALANCED VAGINA IS A HAPPY VAGINA

Newsflash: your vagina has a pH level where all is good and great. If you're a numbers person, it's around 3.5 to 4.5 pH. In case you forgot your grade-school science lessons, pH means how acidic or basic something is, measured on a scale of zero to fourteen. Here's what has similar pH to healthy vaginas: apples, beer, and wine. Your vagina will naturally be at its right pH, especially if you're eating well, drinking lots of fluids, keeping it clean, practicing safe sex, and are generally healthy. But if you mess with your vagina's pH, bad stuff can happen, including infections. Here's a list of some common things that could potentially throw off your vaginal pH:

- fragrance (found in soap, laundry detergent residue, or even tampons)
- certain ingredients in most conventional personal lubricants (see page 220)
- semen
- douching

- wearing wet gym clothes or yoga pants for too long

- poor health and/or poor diet

- hormonal imbalance

Pay careful attention to those and your pH will stay balanced.

Luckily your vagina is home to a lot of good bacteria—the second largest amount of bacteria in a body after the gut, actually. The good bacteria are there to keep things healthy and to help regulate your vagina's pH level by fighting and killing bad bacteria. But sometimes the balance of bacteria is thrown off, and then your pH will also be thrown off. This can lead to infection and inflammation; increased pH can kill off good bacteria, then the bad bacteria can multiply and lead to infections like bacterial vaginosis (see page 37). Balance is key.

VAGINAS ARE NOT UNSCENTED

Vaginas smell. And they're supposed to smell. You know, more or less like your armpits do, but a lot less pungent. As in: no deodorants are needed. You actually have sweat glands down there—why else do you see massive wet stains after a workout?—so of course your vagina smells.

Every vagina has its own unique scent. Chances are you've

had a partner or two comment favorably on your scent and taste before. Odor, even a little funky, can be hot. It's a combination of what bacteria happen to be there and what you eat and how you dress and if you walk around in sweaty workout clothes and how frequently you bathe and pheromones biologically there to attract partners. Yup, smell is biologically linked to reproduction. Factor in if you spray perfume or add creams to mask your personal odor, plus how often you go to the bathroom and how well you wipe.

Want to smell less? Shower. Keep things clean. Avoid too-tight clothes. Wear cotton panties or no panties at all. If it doesn't disturb your sleep, try going commando overnight, especially if you're prone to bacterial or yeast infections. It can get pretty stuffy in moist underwear as you sleep. Change out of sweaty workout clothes soon after working out. And, even though it may seem counterintuitive, avoid scented products, too. They can lead to rashes and infections, which throw off your all-important vaginal pH and harm the good vaginal bacteria. Smell can be a sign your pH is out of whack. So do not douche, whatever you do! Douching can offset the normal flora (bacteria) and predispose you to infection. Your cervical mucus is truly taking care of your vagina; trust it. No need to flush water and irritating perfume up there in an effort to "clean" it. It could even increase your risk of STIs. Keep in mind that scent can change throughout the month depending on where you are in your reproductive cycle. It's typically all within the range of normal. But if something smells really off, like not your normal scent, you'll know it. Then go see your doctor to figure out if something serious is up or if you just forgot a tampon up there last month. It happens more than you'd think!

SELF-CARE

Truly, the vagina is a self-cleaning organ. Your discharge is already doing the internal work for you. On the exterior, your vulva does not need a car wash–esque scenario to be considered clean. Warm water and maybe a washcloth daily—especially when you have your period—is all you need. And get in there—in and around the labia, up under (gently!) that clitoral hood, where vaginal secretions can build up—this is called smegma, or some people refer to it as cheese. If the secretions aren't washed away regularly and they dry out, they can form little hard kernels. It's super easy to rinse off. Also pay attention to that spot between your vagina and your ass; that's important to keep clean. Want a little more cleaning power? Only use mild, unscented soap, preferably made with natural ingredients. Chemicals and perfumes found in many conventional soaps are just too harsh for a vagina, and using them can disturb your vaginal pH and healthy bacteria and may result in skin irritations or even a yeast infection. Many soaps, bodywashes, douches, and vaginal wipes can contain hormone-disrupting

WHAT *IS* FRAGRANCE?

Fragrance sounds like it should be one specific ingredient. But it's actually a word that product makers use as a placeholder for up to five thousand different ingredients both natural and synthetic (some people say less, some people say more)! The specific mix of those ingredients is protected as a trade secret by US regulations. Not knowing what's in your products means you can't make informed choices. Even if consumers can't know what the exact mix is, we do know that typical fragrance chemicals have been linked in studies to everything from hormone disruption to asthma to skin irritation to cancer. So when you see *fragrance* listed on a soap or a bodywash or vaginal wipes or a candle you use to set the mood or even your personal lubricant, mentally translate that as *hidden, possibly toxic, ingredients*.

Even unscented items can contain chemical-masking agents that suppress scent. Using natural products from companies that voluntarily disclose their ingredients is always the best bet, especially if the companies go out of their way to seek third-party certification to back up their claims. But keep in mind that natural scents like essential oils can also be irritating to skin, especially delicate skin. So when using products down there, use caution and care, and always read labels!

When it comes to pads and tampons, many of which are sold scented, ingredient lists can be hard to find. (The US Food and Drug Administration actually doesn't even require these manufacturers to disclose their ingredients!) So look for brands that choose to list their ingredients, and be wary of marketing claims like *fresh scent* or *deodorant*, as these can serve as warnings that the contents of the box are perfumed. There's no amount of perfume that's worth killing off your vagina's good bacteria. For more on feminine care, turn to page 64.

chemicals—not anything you want around your vagina. It's such a sensitive organ. Avoid them—even if they claim to be formulated for pH balance. Remember the vagina is a mucosal membrane. Anything that comes into contact with it can be absorbed into the bloodstream. This is true of skin, too, but things are much more readily absorbed by mucosal membrane. When shopping for cleansers or any products that might come into contact with your vagina, look at the labels on the bottle. Read the ingredients to avoid petrochemicals, harsh surfactants, fragrance, dyes, and questionable preservatives like parabens. If you don't understand or recognize the listed ingredients, do a little research to make sure it's safe to be on and around the most intimate part of your body. For more on what ingredients are best to avoid on and around your vagina, check out Women's Voices for the Earth's comprehensive guide at WomensVoices.org and see page 220.

GROOMING

Beyond showering, a little grooming can help keep things clean. Trimming, waxing, lasering, shaving, sugaring, or whatever form of hair removal you choose can reduce the sweat, odor, and pheromones that can get trapped in pubic hair, especially if yours is on the thick side or if you've got hair between your vagina and your anus. Some people say taking our hair off isn't "natural"; we're supposed to have pubes. Hair is there to protect our bodies and keep them warm. But an upside of going bare, if that's your style of choice, is that we and our partners can really see what our vulvas look like. In all their glory.

Here's the downside of hair removal, either if you DIY or you have someone else do it: when you remove it, your skin can get irritated and inflamed. Ripping or shaving hair from our bodies leaves tiny open wounds in a super moist environment. You know where this is headed . . . those little cuts leave you vulnerable to infections. Wet climates are a perfect growing spot for a whole host of bad bacteria—even staph. As anyone who has ever shaved a bikini line or even their whole vulva knows, ingrown hairs and little pus-filled bumps are the norm. You also increase your risk for STIs if you're sexually active shortly after, say, having your pubes Brazilianed. This is not at all to say don't remove your hair. Just: be aware and be careful. And if you're going bare, make sure you're getting your hair removed in a clean environment.

DIY

If you're doing the hair removal yourself, do it with care! This tends to mean shaving, because it's cheap and fast. But don't be in such a hurry. To avoid the dreaded red bumps, shaving should be done with a sharp, clean, and new razor (never use an old razor—they increase chances of infection) and with whatever products you know work to protect your body from razor burn and ingrown hairs. Not sure what works? Test a few shaving creams or soaps out before denuding yourself entirely, preferably one made from fragrance-free, natural, and otherwise soothing vagina-friendly ingredients. Some people swear by soaking in warm water before shaving. Others swear by exfoliating. By all accounts, you want to shave in the direction your hair grows. After, try to close your pores by using cold water or even ice, and use a soothing product that doesn't contain harsh, irritating ingredients. Some people like witch hazel and, after the pores close, coconut oil. There are all kinds of over-the-counter remedies, too. If you get ingrown hairs or pimples, don't pop them! Warm compresses are an effective and gentler treatment. If you wind up with an infection, get yourself to your doctor.

If dealing with shaving, or the considerable sticky mess of at-home waxing and/or paying the price to get professionally waxed, plus stubble and infections make you want to give up entirely and embrace your natural look, go for it. If the girls of *Broad City* have taught us anything, it's that full bush is making a serious comeback. Or maybe it never went away. To each her own hairdo.

Trimming

It's both low-tech and highly effective (though not so much on the bikini line). Just be very focused when you're maneuvering sharp scissor blades or an electric trimmer around your labia.

Laser

Lasering your hair can be very freeing—if you have the kind of hair and skin that makes you a candidate for this process. Typically you need to have dark hair and light skin, though the technology is constantly evolving, and there are lasers now that work on a wide variety of skin tones. Ask a technician about their lasers and if you can get a patch test done. If you're good to go, it's expensive and time-consuming (until you're done, anyway). And it's permanent. So it's kind of like getting a tattoo: you're stuck with it for life. You might like your pubic hair a certain way today that, in a few years' time, you won't want anymore. So just think it through.

VAGINAL WORKOUTS ARE A THING

The secret to keeping a vagina healthy is the same stuff you already know you need to do for your whole body: eat well, get sleep, drink lots of water, and work out. It's surrounded by muscles, after all. You have to use them, or you'll lose them. It gets happy—the more blood supply to the area helps to keep it alive and vibrant. Normal full-body exercises help keep the pelvic floor in general good shape, but there are also pelvic muscle–

specific workouts that can be done if you find yourself feeling weak down below. This can happen after gaining weight, pregnancy, and childbirth, plus as you age. Generally speaking: using it by having sex should suffice; you don't need to specifically work out the muscles around your vagina—unless you want to.

Kegels

Pelvic floor exercises are actually a proven way to flex love muscles. There is science behind the method, which is basically contracting or squeezing, then relaxing your below-the-belt muscles a few times a day for a set amount of time. You do not, however, need to buy anything like toys or props to work out with. If you'd like to, that's up to you. Kegels can be a bit tedious. For motivation, just keep reminding yourself that learning how to isolate and focus your attention on the muscles around your vagina may help you attain orgasm more easily, intensely, and frequently.

Mula Bandha

This is kind of like yoga Kegels, but also kind of not. If you've ever been to a yoga class, you've probably heard the term, also referred to as *root lock. Mula bandha* is associated with the center of the perineum; for women you basically contract and hold the area at the base of the cervix, though everyone describes it differently. You "lock" it during meditation or while holding poses. Over time, it gets stronger. This can intensify orgasm.

Have Sex and/or Masturbate

Think about all that spasming that happens when you orgasm. Lots of orgasms can strengthen things. It's a muscle, so go ahead and flex it.

If you take to the Internet to find ways to work out your vagina, you might run across suggestions like taking certain herbs or even getting surgery (no way!). Please ignore this information. The questionable herbal pills or cocktails that are supposed to help "tighten" women are mainly bad for you. Walk away. And don't try to lift random heavy things with your vagina, either. Yes, some doctors or physical therapists will suggest adding actual weights to Kegels—depending on your own body's needs—but that's for you and your doctor or physical therapist to discuss.

VISITATION RIGHTS: GET THE MOST OUT OF YOUR OB-GYN APPOINTMENTS

Speaking of doctors, taking your vagina for a yearly visit is an absolute must! Think of this annual trip to the ob-gyn or primary care doctor as a critical part of your overall self-care and wellness. Gynecologists look at vaginas all day long, so it's important to check in with them to make sure yours is happy and healthy. Health care isn't the easiest thing in this day and age, and many of us wind up not even going to the same doctor year after year. Finding an ob-gyn you like and trust is important. You want to be with someone you feel comfortable talking to about random bumps you might have, STI tests, discomfort, smells, and maybe even sharing good news like that you learned how to masturbate and it has changed your life for the better. Even if you don't have a doctor you always see yearly, just make sure you see one! And if you have questions that come up or you want an STI test (see page 166), and it hasn't been a year since your last appointment, you clearly don't have to wait for a yearly. Go visit.

While you're there, it's important to be honest about your sex life—it's information your doctor needs to know to help safeguard your health. Ask any questions you might have about anything you've been thinking about. If you have any concerns about your birth control, speak up. Want to know why your discharge looks a certain way? Show and tell. You're there for a reason, and doctors are a great resource. So use them.

And if you're ever in a situation where your gynecologist is making you feel uncomfortable or like you're not being listened to, ditch that doctor. Yes, they went to medical school and maybe you did not, but no gynecologist should ever make you feel vulnerable or bad. If they do, well, there are plenty of other fish in the sea.

COMMON CONCERNS

There are a lot of things that can go wrong below the belt. Some (cervical cancer) are a lot worse than others (yeast infections). For the not-so-bad stuff, women can often care for their vaginas without a doctor's input, or with minimal input. Here's how to know if and when to make an appointment for the everyday aches, pains, bumps, and burns.

Yeast Infection

Causes: The yeasty beasty is a super common and annoying experience. Three-quarters of all women suffer through it at some point—usually after a round of antibiotics, which can throw the normal balance of bacteria and yeast out of whack. Taking probiotics including acidophilus before, during, and after could help. A typical yeast infection is caused by the organism *Candida albicans*—an overgrowth of the fungus. You know you've got one if you're itching, though some other lovely things can rear their heads, too: burning, discharge (pretty chunky), and pain. It's not technically an STI, because women who aren't sexually active certainly can and do get yeast infections. Still, depending on who you're sleeping with, your yeast infection could pose risks for your partners. While it's hard to pass a yeast infection from a vagina to a penis, women who sleep with women could potentially transmit an infection through shared sex toys or oral sex.

Treatment: All hail antifungal medication; it's over-the-counter stuff! If you're itchy and are sure based on past experience that you have a yeast infection, try treating it yourself with this drugstore staple, which is a lot easier than getting an appointment with your gyno. But if the medicine is not working, you have to go see your doctor. Sometimes what we think is a yeast infection is not actually yeast, or it is yeast but you need something stronger, like an oral med. If you have recurrent yeast infections, that's another reason to go to your doctor. It could be a sign of another illness, including diabetes.

Prevention: Keep your vagina dry! Well, as much as it's possible to keep a pretty wet area dry. Like don't hang around forever in a wet bathing suit or your post–spin class pants. Clean gently, use tampons and pads that don't contain fragrance, and don't wash your underwear in harsh detergents, or the residue could irritate you. There is evidence that probiotics can help preventatively, but please, people, do not put yogurt *in* your vagina. Eat it if you like it, but it's not going to do anything internally for your vaginal health.

Urinary Tract Infection (UTI)

Causes: There are so many ways to get a UTI, especially if you're a woman. We have short urethras (that's the tube that connects your bladder to your pee hole), which means the bacteria does not have to travel far to gain access and infect us. During sexual activity people do a lot of things that can push bacteria—from the mouth, from hands, from the body—into the urethra.

Treatment: Sorry, but drinking tons of water and maybe some cranberry juice isn't going to cut it if you have an infection. You're going to need to see your doctor. They will likely take a urine sample and start you on an antibiotic regimen. They can match the drug to the bacteria that's causing it.

Prevention: Always pee before and after sex! Keep your hands and your genitals and your partners' hands and genitals clean. Always wipe front to back, not back to front. Never ever go from anal to vaginal penetration with fingers, a toy, or a penis without cleaning them off and/or switching to a new condom first. (If you do, you might feel telltale signs of an infection pretty quickly, and will want to call your doctor. If you have no signs of infection—you lucked out this time.) You're more at risk if you're in the "honeymoon" phase of a new relationship when you're really going at it a lot, or if you've gone through a dry spell and are back in bed.

Bacterial Vaginosis (BV)

Causes: Vaginal ecology is a tricky thing. Sometimes when good bacteria decrease and bad bacteria overgrow in your vagina it's no big deal. And then there's bacterial vaginosis. It's very common—two in five women have it, but 84 percent of women don't even realize they do. Basically it can make you smell like fish. And it creates a lot of discharge that can be thin and grayish (that's just a bunch of cells sloughing off). Who wants either? Depending on how bad the imbalance of bad to good bacteria is, it could clear up on its own in a few days, but you know your body. If it's off, it's off.

Treatment: Got the aforementioned symptoms? Head to your doctor to get your vag checked out. They can diagnose you based on a number of things (not all women with BV have either the smell or the discharge) and can treat with antibiotics you swallow or insert in your vagina. BV is not an issue in and of itself, but having it could put you at higher risk when exposed to an STI (including HIV), so you definitely want to treat it. Even if you take your meds, BV is a recurrent infection. That means it can come back, so keep an eye out for it.

Prevention: Keep your vaginal pH in normal range and you won't likely run into BV. Avoid harsh chemicals and fragrances found in many soaps, personal lubricants, and period products. Douching washes out the vagina's good bacteria and so can lead to BV. So don't douche! Other risk factors include smoking (more reasons to never start, or to quit!) and new or multiple sexual partners. Realistically it's not like you're going to give up sex partners. Who would? Just be safe (and protected) out there.

THREE QUESTIONS

1 MY VAGINA HAS ALL KINDS OF LUMPS AND BUMPS AND PIMPLES. WHAT ARE THEY? HOW DO I KNOW IF THEY'RE OK?

Go stand in front of a mirror and stick out your tongue. Use your hands to pull your cheeks so you can really see the inside of them. The skin there is totally bumpy and weird-looking, right? Well, the skin on your inner lips is similar skin. And, yes, it's super lumpy and bumpy and can sometimes look like something is, well, wrong. The majority of the time, nothing is wrong. If something is, you'll likely know. If you have open red sores, itching that won't go away, the kind of lumps that can be felt but not seen, hard bumps that can be seen and felt on the labia or under your pubic hair, if you have things that look like warts or growths, or just really feel off or uncomfortable and you can't tell why, it's time to get to your doctor. Put down the book, pick up the phone, and make an appointment.

A pimple, however, is not a red raw sore. And pimples happen. So do ingrown hairs. You know what those look like because you have had them elsewhere on your body. They're familiar. Just because they're on your vulva does not mean they're cause for alarm. There are plenty of sweat glands down there and it's generally a hot, warm environment. So of course you get pimples. And if you're busily removing pubic hair, of course you get ingrown hairs. Don't pick pimples or ingrown hairs, just as you would not (or try not to) on your face. Warm compresses can help with either; so can freeing an ingrown hair (that means pulling the hair so it's growing outside your skin instead of underneath it, but don't pluck it). Mainly, let these run-of-the-mill skin issues heal on their own. And don't forget to look closely at your vagina from time to time—the better you know it, the more you'll be able to clearly see what's normal for you and what's not.

2 WHAT CAUSES VAGINAL DRYNESS?

Dry skin is a bummer no matter where it is, but in your vag, it can feel like a total insult. One thing that can lead to dryness for sure is not being into the person you're making out with—more reasons to sleep with people you're hot for! But if you're mentally or otherwise aroused and still dry, then it could be a number of things, including hormones (decreased estrogen is responsible for dryness, especially during perimenopause and menopause, after childbirth, or while breastfeeding), psychological stuff (anxiety, fear, stress, and more), and even side effects from a medication you may be on. And don't neglect irritants, like perfume in your tampons and pads or even laundry detergent residue in your underwear—both can be drying. Having penetrative sex when you are dry can be very painful and it can lead to tearing, which could put you at higher risk for STIs. Thankfully there is lube to the rescue (preferably organic, which won't further irritate your vagina)! Even if lube is fixing the immediate issue, it's not fixing the problem long-term. You'll want to get to the roots of what's causing your dryness. If you're going through cancer treatment, which can cause vaginal dryness, you won't have to scratch too far below the surface to figure out that cause, but some things you might not expect can be drying, like cold medicine with an antihistamine or an allergy pill. They dry out your nasal passage as well as your vagina. If you don't feel like you have a good handle on what's causing your own dryness, go see your gyno. They may have a few estrogen-related tricks up their sleeve besides lube. For the mental stuff, a good therapist is always useful.

3 ONCE, WHEN I WAS HAVING SEX, AIR CAME OUT OF MY VAGINA—KIND OF LIKE A FART BUT IN THE WRONG PLACE. WHAT WAS THAT?

Your self-diagnosis is spot-on! That was what's referred to as a queef or a vaginal fart. There's nothing unhealthy or bad for you about it, so no worries there. But unlike a fart fart, it's not gas coming from digestion but rather a pocket of air getting pushed out of the vagina. It won't smell. Usually this means air that was trapped in the curved vaginal canal during sex. Some women say they can actually make themselves queef by using their abs to draw air in—a good party trick but a less-fun experience if you happen to let air out during, say, a yoga class. There isn't one sexual position you can avoid that's most likely to shove air up there. So when you queef, just go with it. There's no need to stop what you're doing, or change rhythms or directions, just keep going on getting it on.

CHAPTER 2

LET IT FLOW:

ALL ABOUT PERIODS

Riding the crimson wave, shark week, Aunt Flo, parting of the red sea . . . let's talk periods. Probably if you're waiting and hoping/praying/begging that you're not pregnant, you're only thinking you want it. Badly. Now! Or maybe you don't want it because it's annoying or painful or disruptive—like if you have a hot date or weekend travel plans or a new pair of jeans. That's pretty much all most of us consider, at least until we hit the phase of life, if we ever do, when we actually *want* to get pregnant. Kind of ironic.

But, how much do you know about how it works? As inconvenient as it can be, the menstrual cycle is actually an exquisitely beautiful and finely tuned system. (Yes, the word *menstrual* is the worst.) Get to know the inner workings and you'll be wowed. It's beyond amazing—an awe-inspiring feat of nature and evolution that can ruin everything from underwear to sheets to your brand-new pair of vintage Levi's. It's undeniably cool even for those of us who slept through human anatomy and had no desire to ever go to med school. Truly.

A period is not just something that happens naturally once a month. After you go through puberty and before you hit menopause, your cycle is *always* happening. That's what *cycle* means. The week (give or take) that you bleed (aka shed the lining of your uterus) is just one part of it. There are about three other weeks when different stuff is going on. Basically the whole thing is about making or not making a baby—and your hormones direct the entire show: your body gets ready to release an egg to be fertilized. The uterus prepares itself to be a home for a fertilized egg. When fertilization doesn't happen, cue the tampons/pads/cup.

This process happens in a few phases. Depending on how regular your cycle is, or if you're on hormonal birth control, it basically breaks down like this: week one is menstruation; week two is when your body prepares to ovulate; week three is ovulation; week four is PMS, if you happen to get it. And, as you've probably guessed from talking to your friends, your mom, and your coworkers, the experience is a little different for every woman. Even your own cycle can vary month to month. Still, there are obviously some general traits most of us share.

- In the first phase of your cycle, which starts just after you get your period, the estrogen in your

Menstruation Cycle

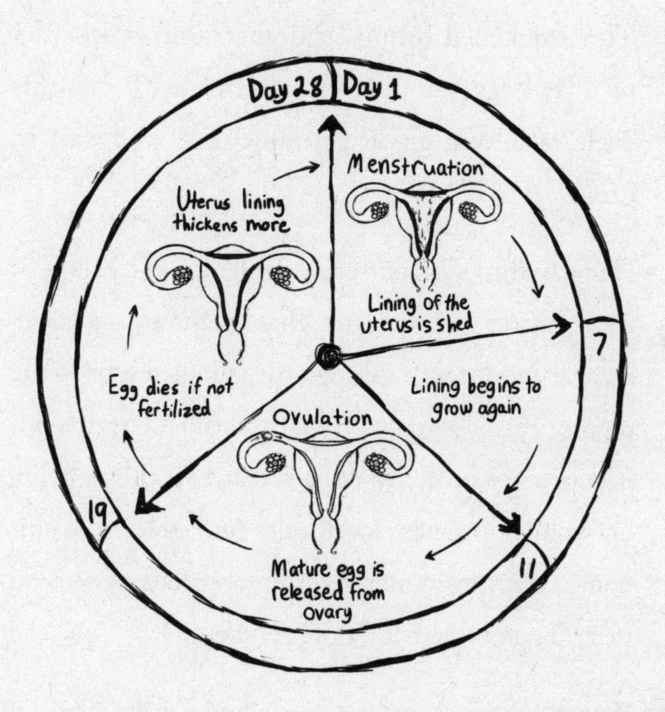

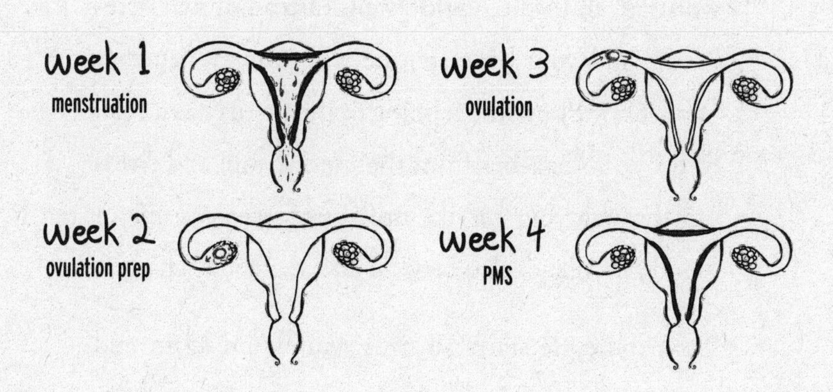

system begins to rise. Estrogen prompts the lining of your uterus to thicken, among other things. This thickened lining (endometrium) is where a fertilized egg, should you wind up with one this cycle, would implant, get nourished, and start to grow.

- Halfway through your cycle, while the thickening is in the works, you ovulate. That means an egg leaves an ovary and travels through the fallopian tube to the uterus. This is when you're most fertile, so watch out if you're not up for making a baby! As this is going on, your hormones, specifically progesterone at this point, are continuing to calibrate your system to make a good home for a pregnancy.

- If your egg never meets a sperm and gets fertilized, it won't attach to the uterine wall. Instead, it will deteriorate and your progesterone will drop. When that happens, the now-thick lining of the uterus has no job to do, so it detaches from the uterine wall and sheds out through your cervix, into your vagina—a mix of blood and tissue, plus cervical and vaginal discharge.

- Then the cycle starts all over again. And again and again and again. These details are obviously just the *very* basics. If the topic fascinates you, Google is your friend. It's easy to learn more about.

A cycle is on average twenty-eight days, and ovulation tends to happen around day fourteen. But things vary. Cycles can range in length and duration. They can be twenty-five days or thirty-two days. Some women change month to month and just never know when, exactly, they're going to get their period. Some months your period will be heavier than others. Some women bleed more than others. The amount of blood is usually related to hormones. If you're on hormonal birth control, chances are your periods are lighter than they'd be if you weren't, or you may not even get a period. The amount you bleed can also change as you age, including after childbirth; the huge hormonal shifts that happen in those nine months can have lasting effects, including differences in your flow. Not all women experience this—some see no increased monthly bleeding after a first pregnancy but then a big shift after a second pregnancy, and so on. And, in your late thirties, as estrogen, egg quality, and fertility begin to decline, your flow can change again. Another time flow likely changes is as you approach menopause, when you stop having periods entirely, during a phase called perimenopause when your hormones fluctuate a lot. Sometimes you'll produce too much or too little estrogen or too much or too little progesterone. This can lead to heavy and inconsistent bleeding, shortened or prolonged cycles, new-to-you or different PMS symptoms, and, eventually, irregular cycles. Our adviser Dr. Nathalie Feldman explains it's all about the balance between these two hormones, not their absolute values. That's what causes the lining to thicken or periods to become irregular.

At any age, period durations vary. Some women only have them for a few days; some women are at it for a week or more. It's pretty standard for young women just starting their cycles to have irregular cycles or even to skip periods. It takes a while for a body to mature to having regular cycles. If things are really irregular or you have not had a period in months, a doctor's visit is in order. Sometimes gynecologists will even prescribe progesterone to bring on a period if you've skipped more than three months and you're not pregnant.

There's a pretty broad range of what is considered medically normal when it comes to periods. Try tracking yours month to month on a calendar or use a period and ovulation tracker app like Clue so you have a sense of what's "normal" for you. Then share your tracked information with your gynecologist at your yearly checkup, or more frequently if you have concerns. Periods can be thought of as a vital sign—they can show us and our doctors what's happening in our bodies. They may even show signs of disease our doctors can "read." For example, heavy bleeding may signal that there's an imbalance of hormones. Some young women with really heavy periods may even be diagnosed with bleeding disorders that have gone undetected until this milestone of puberty. Later in life, knowing the history of how often you get your period and how regular it is can show you—and your doctor—what's up with your fertility, if that's something you want to know.

PERIOD MANAGEMENT

As fascinating as the female reproductive system is, it's pretty much impossible to get awe-inspired when you're doubled over in pain, bloated, sore, and clutching your heating pad like it's your lifeline. Listen up! There's *no* reason to suffer just because you're a woman. Got pain? Seek help! There are a zillion ways to reduce this joy of being female—from natural to medical solutions. Some work really well, some less well; it all depends on your body and your needs. If you're more uncomfortable than you'd like to be and nothing is working—and especially if you're in so much pain you're missing school or work or drinks with your friends—check in with your doctor for ideas you may not be thinking of. When it comes to cramps, it takes a village.

PREMENSTRUAL SYNDROME (PMS)

PMS is a real thing. Here's the deal: the hormones working our systems like puppet masters to create our cycles also affect many other aspects of our nervous systems, including certain cells in our brains, which can change your mood, making you irritable as well as exhausted. You know how sometimes it feels like you're losing your mind and then you get your period and a few days later you're back to yourself and good to go? This is all normal. Thanks, hormones. Some of us get PMS way worse than others. If yours is totally debilitating, you'll want to partner up with your doctor for help. Premenstrual syndrome is also in dire need of a new name, because what's this *pre* thing? Yes, it kicks in shortly before you get your period, when your progesterone drops, but it can last for a little while, like well into the beginning of your period.

Your hormones are also at fault for the fact that you're bloated and feeling like a sausage. They make your body swell and retain fluids. Some say being bloated is more of a feeling than an actual amount of water, though others report seeing water weight as pounds on the scale month to month. Scales don't lie. Neither do your straining pants. Thankfully water weight cycles down as quickly as it cycles up, so try not to take it personally, especially if you're feeling moody. It will soon be gone.

To add insult to injury, you may also be bloated from gas. Hormones can affect your gut, changing how your digestion functions, which is why you may experience constipation and/or diarrhea leading up to your period. Some women even report both! Such a delight. Again, this too shall pass.

Since there are receptors to progesterone and estrogen on other tissues in our bodies beyond the gut, period symptoms are really system-wide. Obviously another typical area of bloat is breasts. Some women have to wear entirely different bra sizes toward the end of their cycle and just before they get their periods. Receptors in breast tissue get stimulated then produce fluid shifts at this time. It's basically an expansion of your milk ducts and can leave you really sore and tender, especially in the second half of your cycle. Once you're feeling this boob pain, if your cycles are pretty regular, you know you're about to get your period. Not everyone gets this pain, formally known as cyclical mastalgia, and some of us feel it way worse than others. Breast tissue is usually denser and bumpier at this stage of the game. Don't let those lumps scare you, but do track them. They should change with hormonal fluctuations. If they don't, go visit your doctor so they can take a look.

The fatigue you're likely experiencing can come from several factors, including if your sleep is being interrupted by painful PMS symptoms. Working out, one of the most effective ways to mitigate PMS symptoms, can usually help tire you enough to sleep through the night. But you could also be anemic. If you're really suffering from exhaustion every month, it may be worth doing a blood test at your doctor's office, and if you're low in iron or your blood count is low, then adding iron-rich foods and maybe even a supplement to your diet could help.

CRAMPS

No amount of sore breasts, fatigue, and gassiness can hold a candle to cramps. They. Are. The. Worst. Don't get them? Lucky you. Get them? So sorry. Here's what cramps are: they're your uterus contracting to move its thickened lining out and, once it has shed, to stop the bleeding. There is a familial component to them—often if your mom gets cramps, you might, too. But that's not always the case. There are certain anatomic issues that can increase painful cramping, like endometriosis, which is when part of the lining of the uterus grows outside it. That's especially unpleasant. Doctors can work with patients who have it to find solutions—everything from hormone suppression to surgery. (Yes, *Girls* fans, this is what Lena Dunham has struggled with.) Women who have not had a baby are more likely to have cramps. The going theory is that after the uterus is stretched out by the growing baby, the muscle and maybe the nerves are less apt to be painful when contracting. But that's of no consolation when you're cramping.

PMS MANAGEMENT

There are so many ways to make your period discomfort a less painful and exhausting experience. They range from diet changes to medications. If you can get results without using medication, that's fabulous. But don't shy away from meds and grit through pain month after month, year after year because you prefer to be natural. Start with food changes to see if you feel better. If not, you can try herbs or over-the-counter meds. But check with your doctor first as some of them have side effects or other potentially harmful things that may not be immediately apparent.

HEALTHY LIVING

Just before a period and during the first few days, a lot of women prefer to laze around and binge-eat ice cream or potato chips or both. Sorry, but you have to fight against this. Eating well, getting lots of fiber, avoiding salty and sugary stuff, drinking lots of water, getting ample sleep, and working out are all scientifically proven to combat PMS. They will make you feel better even if you don't want to do them with every fiber of your being. There are studies that prove that endorphins released from working out help the very same receptors in your brain that alter your mood when dealing with PMS, especially right before you get your period. So get up and get moving. Take a walk. Do some deep breathing or yoga to reduce stress and boost energy. Light, healthy meals will make you feel better than foods that make you cramp or bloat even more than you already are. Avoiding foods that give you quick short-lived energy spikes will help with overall fatigue—you want to keep your blood sugar balanced. Studies also show that lowering caffeine intake can decrease breast pain. This may seem like a bad idea, especially if you suffer from crazy fatigue right before your period, but while caffeine might provide temporary relief, it's not always the answer. Exercising and eating iron-rich foods, as mentioned, should help more than coffee. That said, when you're feeling your worst, maybe you don't want to add a coffee withdrawal headache to your list of ailments. Fair enough. Besides, it's always easier to adhere to a plan that involves a few simple, positive changes rather than forcing yourself to give up what you like or rely on. Speaking of, reducing or giving up alcohol can also help with PMS. Just do what's reasonable for you, keeping in mind that pushing yourself a little in a direction you might not want to go (e.g., your gym clothes) will actually make you feel better.

HEAD EAST!

Chinese medicine has been used to treat menstrual problems for thousands of years—everything from irregular cycle to no cycle to midcycle bleeding to migraines to cramps. Dr. Jill Blakeway, a doctor of acupuncture and Chinese medicine, and a clinical herbalist who founded the awesome YinOva Center in New York City, calls PMS a "poor response to a hormonal transition." Some women feel like they have "dropped off a cliff" when their progesterone decreases. She works with patients to smooth out these hormonal transitions. "There are a lot of imbalances that are subtle but have profound effects that do well with Chinese herbs. We get great results," she says.

Here are six things she suggests for anyone with PMS.

1. **GET REGULAR EXERCISE.** It moves the chi and blood and smooths transition.

2. **EAT CRUCIFEROUS VEGETABLES.** Broccoli, kale, cauliflower, and all their cousins contain an active compound called DIM, which helps with estrogen imbalance.

3. **PRIORITIZE HEALTHY FATS.** This means olive and coconut oils, omega-3s, and the like.

4. **TAKE XIAO YAO WAN.** This herbal formula has been used for hundreds of years to treat PMS, and it's widely available for purchase. It helps with the hormonal transition and supports the liver as it confronts estrogen. Blakeway calls it "miraculous."

5. **TROUBLESHOOT SYMPTOMS WITH VITAMINS.** Irritable? Take B_6. Sore breasts? Try vitamin E. For bloating you want magnesium. If you're feeling weepy, try calcium. One quick word of caution when it comes to vitamins: always make sure to take the appropriate amount. Many vitamins (e.g., B_6 and E) and elements (e.g., magnesium and calcium) have a threshold above which toxicity can occur, so be careful not to take too much.

6. **TRY SEED CYCLING.** This involves taking ground pumpkin and flax seed daily during the follicular phase of your cycle until you ovulate; the theory here is that they help you metabolize estrogen, which rules this phase. After ovulation you switch to sesame and sunflower seeds. Blakeway says they have nutrient precursors to the progesterone, which dominates this phase.

GET WARM

Heat is a no-brainer way to soothe period aches and pains—both PMS and cramps. Heating pads, hot-water bottles, baths, hot tubs—whatever you've got, it's all good. Put your warm dog or cat on your lap! Surround yourself with warmth and chill.

ACUPUNCTURE

Great news: cramps are a relatively straightforward ailment for a licensed acupuncturist to treat. In Chinese medicine, cramps are considered to be caused by poor blood flow, according to Dr. Blakeway, so an acupuncturist will work on triggering adequate circulation. Once circulation is fixed, and depending on how a woman reacts to the treatment, cramps should not be an issue going forward. As in, it should work to actually solve the problem, not as a Band-Aid, like a painkiller.

MEDICINAL MEASURES

First up, there are over-the-counter painkillers. But you have to know when to use them. Cramps are caused by prostaglandins, substances you produce and release during your period to give the signal to the uterus to contract. Anti-inflammatory meds like ibuprofen can block or reduce the production of prostaglandins, so in order for them to be most effective, it's best to take them before the prostaglandins are produced, not once you're already feeling crampy. So while you always want to be careful to never overmedicate, if you're trying to stave off cramps, take your meds nice and early. Bonus: some say that ibuprofen taken before you start bleeding will also decrease the amount of blood you shed. Still other women report it makes them bleed longer.

Depending on what state you live in, you may prefer medical marijuana to drugstore painkillers, though it's clearly not an option if it's illegal where you live or you need to drive or work. If you're in California, you might even be able to get your hands on some of the cannabis-infused creams, tinctures, and rubs made by the actress Whoopi Goldberg, all said to help with cramping and other uterine fun.

HORMONAL BIRTH CONTROL

For women who really suffer from PMS and cramps, hormonal birth control can be a very useful solution. The hormonal IUD, the implant, the shot, the patch, and the pill all make the lining of the uterus thinner, which means periods are lighter. Depending on the method you start using, it may take a moment to achieve this desired result, and there may even be spotting or more bleeding at first. If you're on the pill, it basically suppresses your own cycle—what you'd produce yourself—and creates its own cycle with lower doses of hormones, to boot. This can result in decreased cramps (the pill keeps those prostaglandins in check) and decreased breast pain. You can even use birth control to get rid of periods entirely. If you're on the pill, you do this by not taking the placebo pills and taking the active ones back-to-back. If you use the ring, you would insert a new one back-to-back instead of removing it for a week for a period. And so on. Not getting a period can be especially useful for women who bleed so heavily they become anemic. Using birth control to get rid of your period is not for everyone, and it should only be embarked upon with input from your doctor. There are many women who feel strongly that it just can't be OK not to get a period, who are used to the rhythm and ritual. Some women don't like the idea psychologically. If you're sexually active and not interested in getting pregnant, being able to see actual monthly evidence that you're not with child can be a big relief. Still, other women adore the freedom. Your body, your choice. Keep in mind that while hormonal birth control could be just the thing for managing your PMS, it can bring on other undesirable side effects (see chapter four). Consider the full picture and how it will impact your overall health.

PERIOD SEX

Some people love it, some people hate it. Hopefully, whatever camp you're in, you have a partner who agrees with your feelings on having sex while you're flowing. If you're both into it, great. Periods are, after all, just bodily fluid. You know what else is bodily fluid? Ejaculate. So what's the big deal? There's a lot of potential upside: orgasm contracts the uterus, which can help soothe cramps and may even hasten your flow and shorten your period. And you have built-in extra lubrication. Just plan for the mess. Use old sheets or a dark towel underneath you. Obviously tampons are no good for vaginal intercourse (with a penis or a toy), so make sure to remove yours before you get going. You could try a disposable menstrual cup if yours can be worn during penetration (not all can—read package instructions) or oral sex to reduce flow in the moment. Remember: cups are not birth control, nor do they protect against STIs. Condoms make an awesome barrier, too, and can be worn in tandem with a cup.

Speaking of condoms, if you are going to have penis-in-vagina sex or oral sex when you're having your period, you definitely want to take all the necessary precautions to protect you and your partner.

Blood can transmit various STIs. And because, yes, you can still get pregnant if you have sex during your period! It's a common fallacy that too many people believe: you can't get pregnant when you have your period. Your first day of menstruation starts your new cycle. If you're pretty regular, you won't likely release an egg for two weeks, but cycle lengths vary! It's hard to know. What if you get your period every twenty-one days instead of every twenty-eight? You're likely to ovulate much sooner. You might be a day seven or nine ovulator. A sperm and an egg can hang around before implanting. So if you're on day three and you're a day seven ovulator, then theoretically you can get pregnant. Sperm can live inside you for up to five days. If you have sex toward the end of your period, do the math. The probabilities aren't huge, but it's possible. Wrap it up.

Of course, period sex doesn't have to mean penis-in-vagina sex, and it doesn't have to equal oral sex. There is plenty to do sexually that will involve no contact with uterine lining, if you'd like to avoid it. Get creative.

PERIOD PRODUCTS

The average woman sheds several ounces of fluid per month. Obviously different women flow varying amounts. So maybe a few ounces sounds like way too little or far too much. If you're using hormonal birth control you may have very light bleeding. Whatever amount you've got, there is a whole host of ways to capture those ounces: pads, tampons, reusable cups, and even reusable underwear. Your preference is your preference, but get to know your choices. Don't just grab the first box you see and give it no further thought. Why? Your vagina is one of the most absorbent parts of your body, which makes it especially vulnerable to harmful substances. Chemicals or substances placed into your vagina can be absorbed through your skin (here it's your mucosal membrane) and go directly into your bloodstream. Some chemicals even go straight to your uterus and stay there. It's important to educate yourself on what you're putting inside you—what it's made of and how to use it. Unfortunately, to date, there has not been one long-term study done on how chemicals found in many mainstream tampons affect women's bodies over time. It's totally wild. The National Institutes of Health (NIH) only started vaginal research in 1992. Better late than never.

While no specific studies have been done on the impact chemicals typically found in most period products—pesticide residue, dioxins, and various petrochemicals—can have in an environment as absorbent as the vagina, it's good common sense to consider them. Why not actively seek out products that minimize your exposure to potentially damaging substances? Here's the frustrating catch: learning about materials and exact ingredients in period care is easier said than done. Despite the fact that tampons (but not pads and liners) are regulated by the US Food and Drug Administration (FDA) as a class II medical device, the agency does not currently require tampon manufacturers to list the ingredients in their products. This is ridiculous, especially considering that tampons are such a widely used form of period care in the United States. The average woman uses around eleven thousand tampons over her lifetime, for approximately forty years. In the absence of totally transparent information on an ingredient list, here's a quick checklist of what to look out for when trying to understand what period products work best for you:

Absorbency ABCs

Read packaging labels for absorbency levels on pads and tampons or sizes for menstrual cups. For tampons, absorbency is standardized brand to brand, and regulated by the FDA. A super means the same thing no matter what brand you're buying. You want to match your product to your flow. If you're on the last day and things are light, don't get lazy and stick a super tampon up there and just change it twelve hours later. That could lead to a number of issues, some of them (toxic shock syndrome, see page 79) a whole lot worse than others. Pulling out a dry tampon when your flow is super light can cause tearing of tissue, making you more at risk for STIs, too. So use small tampons for light days. Or skip tampons entirely and use a liner or wear absorbent underwear instead. And while it's probably OK to wear the correct absorbency tampon overnight for about eight hours, you don't want to wear it longer than that. Changing it more often is ideal. Wearing pads? Change regularly—depending on your flow, but at least every eight hours.

Reusable Versus Disposable

Some people like to see just how much flow they're producing in a month. For them, a reusable menstrual cup is the bomb. Another reason people like reusable period products such as the cup and washable cloth pads is environmental; reusable items produce less waste. If you're interested in eco-friendly options other than reusables, there are organic cotton products (organic agriculture is better for Mother Earth than conventional) and applicator-free tampons, which involve less packaging. Prefer applicators? Choose bioplastic, which comes from a renewable resource and may even be recyclable (postrinse), depending on your municipality. Petroleum-based plastic applicators are not biodegradable and create a fair amount of waste. If price is an issue, keep in mind that while reusable items will cost more up front, they likely will save money over time. Reusable cloth pads come in a variety of fabrics, from fleece to hemp to cotton, and some are better to have around your vulva than others in terms of breathability and potential bacterial growth—the more natural the fabric, the better. They come in varying thicknesses—super useful for overnight—and can be washed over and over again for months and even years.

Fragrance

We've already discussed how *fragrance* is a word that's actually a placeholder for a mix of possibly hundreds of chemicals that make up any given scent—and are protected by our government as a trade secret (see page 27). And we've already spelled out that typical chemicals used in most fragrances are known hormone (endocrine) disruptors. And you already know that scented items, even if you will never know what ingredients, exactly, they contain, can lead to things like yeast infections and bacterial vaginosis. Also, they can make you itchy and rashy because fragrances are known to contain numerous irritant and allergenic chemicals. And yet fragranced tampons and pads are a thing. Despite the fact that 15 to 30 percent of the general population reports at least some sensitivity to chemicals used to make tampons fragrant. Guess what? The American College of Obstetricians and Gynecologists recommends against using scented pads and tampons. You don't need "fresh"-scent tampons or pads. You smell just fine. And you don't deserve to itch or get an infection from a secret formula of fragrance chemicals. Menstrual flow is no different than daily vaginal discharge when it comes to bacteria. You do not need deodorant tampons, and they're more likely to harm you than help you. Concerned? Just wash yourself well—with mild, fragrance-free soap. The end.

Materials Matter

No matter what you're using—tampons, a cup, pads—you always need to know what your period products are made of so you can avoid petrochemicals, pesticide, bleach, fragrances, and dioxin residues, and anything that could irritate or otherwise harm your vagina. Think about it: you're placing this thing—for hours a day, days a month, months a year for years and years—next to your most intimate and highly absorbent skin. When you're considering what to buy, ask yourself if studies about the safety of the materials in it are available. Are the materials man-made or are they natural? What sort of fillers or residues are in there? Are you comfortable using plastic—even high-grade generally-considered-safe plastic—in an acidic environment for that long? Give materials the kind of consideration your vagina deserves. If you don't know the answers to these questions for the products you are currently using, ask the manufacturer to give you more information.

WHAT PERIOD PRODUCTS ARE MADE OF

Even if you've been getting your period for years, don't skip over this section. You'll likely learn something new that will help you make an informed choice about your period products.

The Classics: Disposable Pads and Tampons

Many brands make pads out of a blend of synthetic fibers, cotton, wood pulp, and other (undisclosed) additives. Tampons are typically made using a mix of rayon, polyester, artificial fibers, and dyes, plus plastic applicators and sometimes fragrance. But not to worry! There are alternatives. There are many 100 percent organic cotton options to use instead. If you're already eating organic food or using natural skin care, you likely know a little about the varied benefits of organic agriculture—for the environment, for farm workers, and for your body. For something as absorbent and intimate as vaginas are, organic is a great option to choose if you can.

Rayon

Although rayon is originally derived from a naturally occurring cellulose, the process for creating it is so extensive and chemically intensive that by the time it's produced into a fiber, it's no longer considered natural. So it's usually classified as a manufactured fiber. Its manufacture is notoriously bad for the environment and the resulting product can contain a number of chemical residues including dioxins (see box, page 71) from the bleaching process. Rayon can also increase the risk of toxic shock syndrome (more on that on page 79). And yet it remains in tampons because it's quite absorbent.

Cotton: Conventional Versus Organic

Tampons and pads often contain cotton, usually as part of a cotton-rayon blend, though some products are 100 percent cotton. If you're not up on conventional cotton crop production—and most of us are not—here's what you need to know: it's one of the world's most sprayed crops. The numbers tracking this sort of thing vary year to year, but basically cotton growers use approximately 10 percent of all agricultural chemicals worldwide and 25 percent of the world's total supply of insecticides. Some farmers use cotton genetically modified to be resistant to certain pests and may be able to spray less. The World Health Organization (WHO) has classified many of these pesticides as "extremely or highly hazardous." The manufacture of many of the kinds of pesticides and herbicides used on cotton crops releases dioxin (see box, page 71) into the environment. Dioxin can also be left in the product as a contaminant. Then that product gets used to make your tampon. Five of the nine most commonly used cotton pesticides have been identified as possible human carcinogens. Others are known to damage the nervous system and/or are suspected of disrupting the

DIOXIN

Here's the deal: dioxins are a class of chemicals, toxic at low levels, that have been designated persistent organic pollutants. This means they take a long time to break down once they're in the environment. In 1994, the Environmental Protection Agency (EPA) declared that dioxins are known to cause cancer in animals, and likely to trigger the disease in people. Because the majority of cotton, wood pulp, and rayon found in pads and tampons are bleached with some form of chlorine, they can contain low levels of dioxins. The FDA says this low contamination poses no risk to humans, which contradicts statements from the EPA saying there is no "acceptable level" of exposure to dioxins.

Dioxins are persistent in the environment and in people, and can accumulate in bodily tissues with repeated exposures. They accumulate in the food chain, mostly in fatty tissues, and the majority of human exposure is through edibles, mainly meat and dairy products. Though the EPA does not spell this out, women who use some conventional tampons monthly for about forty years are also in repeated contact. Independent tests done by Arnold Schecter, a professor of environmental sciences at the University of Texas School of Public Health at Houston and a specialist on dioxin's health effects, have found detectable levels of dioxins in the products of a dozen major tampon brands. And, according to Peter deFur, a researcher with the Center for Environmental Studies at Virginia Commonwealth University in Richmond, Virginia, if "a sensitive area such as the endometrium is exposed to dioxin, there would be a near 100 percent absorption of the chemical. It crosses membranes. It is taken up, transported, and stored." At the moment, there's no science available to address what happens when vaginal or endometrial tissue is directly exposed to dioxins. But certainly there is reason to be concerned; it's incredibly sensitive and hormonally responsive tissue. Being exposed to a dioxin orally or otherwise just isn't the same thing. As the scientists continue to gather the data, it seems the best choice for a healthy vagina is organic cotton bleached without chlorine, which is free of production-related dioxins.

body's hormonal system. Cotton pesticides have been linked to infertility, neurological dysfunction, and developmental defects. Once inside living things, including human beings, their persistence means they can still be measured decades after the original exposure occurred. This is bad news for more than your vagina; these chemicals pollute groundwater and soil and harm aquatic wildlife.

This all sounds overwhelmingly scary, but there's a super easy fix to avoid being associated with conventional cotton production and what's potentially harmful in the end product. If you'd like to use tampons and pads, try to choose those made with certified organic cotton. By law, it can't be sprayed with nonorganic pesticides and insecticides, so it's far less likely than conventional cotton to contain residues of harsh chemicals you don't want in your vagina.

Bleaching

The majority of cotton and wood pulp found in period products gets bleached. Bleaching can be done several ways. One process creates by-products and pollutants including dioxins. Thanks to widespread concern about dioxins and other pollutants created by bleaching with pure chlorine over the years, manufacturers have developed two alternative processes: elemental chlorine-free (ECF) bleaching and totally chlorine-free bleaching (TCF). ECF uses chlorine dioxide instead of chlorine bleach (sodium hypochlorite) to whiten fibers and was widely adopted by the industry after a 1998 ruling by the EPA required pulp mills in the United States to reduce their production of chlorinated pollutants. ECF reduces the release of chlorinated pollutants by more than a factor of ten, which is good, but it does not eliminate them. TCF bleaching does eliminate the release of chlorinated pollutants by replacing chlorine entirely with an oxygen bleach like hydrogen peroxide. Since no chlorine is used, no dioxins are formed, released, or remain as residue in the finished product. That makes TCF bleaching the safest. It's generally used by manufacturers of organic cotton products. Look for it; your vagina deserves it.

New Kids on the Block: Cups and Period Underwear

There has arguably not been a whole lot of innovation on the period-products front, but the past decade or so has brought a few cool options into the realm of tampons and pads. Some of them aren't technically new (menstrual cups have been around for more than eighty years!) but are currently having a real moment, so there are more and newer options on the market. If you're not a fan of getting all up in your period blood, or would prefer to keep your exposure to it at a minimum, a reusable cup or period underwear might not be for you. But if you don't mind blood, there's a lot to be said for these items.

Reusable products drastically reduce waste and put less strain on your wallet over time.

Cups

Reusable menstrual cups are usually made either from medical-grade silicone (a must if you have a latex allergy) or natural rubber. They come in a few sizes—usually one for women who have not yet had kids, and another for those who have. You choose one based on the manufacturer's specs and your knowledge of your own body. When you have your period, you can wear a cup for ten to twelve hours, following the specific product's instructions. Basically it fills up and you just take it out and rinse it off a few times a day, then reinsert. Some women love that using a cup makes them that much more intimately involved with their cycle—you can actually see the amount of fluid you're producing versus not being able to really tell from a used tampon or pad. By all accounts, once you get the hang of things, there are very few leaks. Though removal can be messy until you get good at it. Some women like to do this with disposable gloves. Whatever works!

When it comes to cleaning, you have to wash cups the week you have your period. Some cup brands sell washes specifically for their products and list on their websites what not to use if you don't buy their wash—or else you risk damaging the cup. Read all ingredients in whatever you use to wash the cup, including the washes formulated for cups, to see if you deem it safe to use on something so intimate. As always, avoid anything fragranced. Some brands suggest boiling cups when you're finished with your period and storing them a specific way until the next month, others don't. Cups, treated well, are super durable. Some brands say their cups can last ten years! Others suggest replacing yearly. Vaginal pH and cleaning agents will shorten a cup's life span. You need to look at it for signs of wear and tear from time to time. And, again, it depends on the brand and the material—so follow the instructions that came with your cup.

Another big benefit women report about their cups is that, because they collect rather than absorb menstrual fluid, they don't disrupt the natural moisture balance of the vagina. For some women this translates to less cramping and less potential for messing up that all-important vaginal pH. If you're a fan of period sex, keep in mind that cups usually need to be removed before penetration, so follow manufacturer instructions there, too. There are now also plastic disposable cups that look kind of like a diaphragm that can be worn while you're at it, and keep blood out of your vagina. Neither disposable nor reusable cups are contraceptives. But you knew that, right?

Period Underwear

If free bleeding into a special pair of reusable washable period panties (what up, Thinx?) gives you pause, you're not alone.

WATER WORKS

You know how if you go swimming or even take a bath, it feels like your period stops? It doesn't—really—so don't go tampon-free to the pool. Basically what happens is the pressure of the water may keep blood from flowing outside your vagina, but you're for sure still bleeding and there's no promise it won't come out as you move around or get into and out of the body of water. It's a gravity/physics thing. Also, while we're on the subject of swimming, feel free to hit the ocean when you have your period. Sharks won't smell your blood and come seek you out. That's BS.

And it's not really your fault. Since the moment we learn about periods, we're taught how to trap that liquid, not let it flow, and certainly not let it seep into underwear instead of lining those underwear to protect them. If you can get over the mental hump and give a pair of these a try, you may find you love them. Or you may find them an awesome backup for a tampon or even a cup if you're worried about leakage on a heavy-flow day. The surprisingly thin fabric used in period panties is specifically manufactured to be moisture-wicking, absorbent enough to capture several tampons' worth of fluid (depending on the style of underwear), and leak-resistant. Care is pretty simple—you rinse, then wash with your regular laundry. They're a little pricey up front, but if you treat them well, they last for a while and will definitely save you money in the long run. Of all the period inventions in the last few years, we're big fans of these undies.

THREE QUESTIONS

1 I HAVE BAD PERIODS AND I WANT TO GO ON THE PILL TO GET RID OF THEM. BUT I HEAR IF YOU GO ON THE PILL, YOU WON'T WANT TO HAVE SEX. IS THAT TRUE?

There are plenty of women who say their sex drive feels reduced when on hormonal birth control. Basically when you take the pill, you "turn off" your own cycle and you don't ovulate. Ovulation is often associated with increased desire—that's biological. When we release an egg, our libido shoots up; that's what propagates our species. Our bodies *want* sperm then. So, if you suppress that process, then libido will be negatively affected. It's harder to actively want action when your midcycle surge isn't telling you to look for it. Also, the pill can actually decrease free testosterone in your body, so that could be the culprit. Another thing that can tamp down your desire is if you're taking the pill back-to-back and don't get your period at all. Anecdotally, some women say the visual of seeing they're not pregnant is what gets them emotionally excited to have sex.

But here's the thing: this isn't always the case for all women. Some people report decreased sex drive because they're too afraid of getting pregnant. For them, there's such a huge mental relief to being on the pill that it actually increases sex drive. All of this goes down to the fact that, biology be damned, the biggest organ of libido is, after all, the brain—research backs this up. There are just so many psychological factors that influence our desire. Honestly, you won't know how you will feel until you're on the pill. The good news is you can always go right back off it if you don't like how it's affecting your libido.

2 WHAT ARE THE CLOTS WHEN I HAVE MY PERIOD, AND WHAT'S UP WITH ALL THE DIFFERENT COLORS—I THOUGHT BLOOD IS RED!

Clots or clumps and a period that ranges from rusty to dark red and pretty much any color in between are both totally normal. Remember, what's coming out of you is uterine lining, not just blood like what's in your veins or what you see if you cut yourself shaving. The colors tend to vary with amount of flow and age—it gets darker and browner on your lightest days, which come both at the beginning and especially the end of your period. The dark color can also mean it's older blood. Bright red usually happens in the middle of your period when your flow is heaviest and fastest, and it's the newer uterine lining. Some women with heavy and fast periods only flow red. The clumpy stuff is usually just tissue or menstrual flow with discharge. You know how your blood clots when you cut yourself? Well, during your period there are anticoagulants released that allow your flow to, well, flow. Sometimes if you're bleeding quickly, it can still clot a little. It's nothing to worry about. The only time you need to feel concerned is if you're gushing like a fire hose and soaking tampons or pads at an alarming rate. Then you'll want to call your doctor.

3 WHAT'S THE DEAL WITH TSS?

That's toxic shock syndrome and it's a super rare but potentially fatal disease with some truly horrible symptoms. It's caused by a bacterial toxin and is associated with tampon use. Young women are more likely to get TSS than older women. If you don't die from it, you could wind up having to amputate limbs. But hang on, there's good news: if you're changing your tampon regularly, you don't really need to worry about TSS. Incidences of TSS are incredibly few and far between. They appear to have peaked in 1980, according to the Centers for Disease Control and Prevention (CDC), and have been falling since. This is thanks, in part, to increased FDA regulation of tampon materials (the kinds that are the most ideal breeding grounds for TSS are no longer permitted for use) and the standardization of tampon absorbency across brands. There has also been an increase in education and labels, including warning labels on tampon packaging. To protect yourself against TSS, wear a tampon that is the lowest possible absorbency level for your flow and don't leave it in for longer than you should—change it every four to eight hours. Synthetic fibers can be more absorbent than 100 percent cotton but they can also produce toxins from menstrual bacteria, making the risk for TSS higher. (Synthetic [i.e., noncotton tampons] used to be made from superabsorbent polyester, carboxymethylcellulose, polyacrylate rayon, and viscose rayon, all ideal breeding grounds for TSS. Today only viscose rayon is still permitted for use.) Whatever you choose to wear, always follow package directions and never wear a tampon between periods. For overnights, if you're willing to wear pads, period underwear, or a menstrual cup, go for it. If not, use the least-absorbent tampon that works for your flow and don't forget it's in there! (Happens to the best of us.) Meanwhile, if you ever experience itching with a sudden high fever, red sores, headaches, muscle aches, vomiting, your skin flaking off, dizziness, or smelling something really off, call your doctor—pronto!

CHAPTER 3

YOU DO YOU: A GUIDE TO SELF-PLEASURE

There has never been a better time to have a vagina. There's so much focus on and awareness about pleasure and orgasm right now, and to say we're excited about it is the understatement of the century. Women are more comfortable than ever talking about turn-ons and turn-offs and experiencing their own bodies and taking care of them. So here's a friendly reminder: self-love *is* self-care. And it's high time for some self-love.

If you're not already masturbating, take this as a call to arms: get to it! There are so many reasons to go do you, and the first and best reason is that it feels really, really supremely good. Spend time getting to know what you like and what works and what results in all the feels and, hopefully, eventually an orgasm. Not that you have to—take all the time you want stroking yourself with no goal in sight, as long as it feels great. This is not so you can go make a partner happy, this is for *you*. Because as every sex expert says, every time anyone brings up orgasm, the vast majority of women don't get there from penetration alone. So it's a good idea to learn how you personally get there. Once you've perfected what sends you over the edge, it will be easier to replicate in real time with someone else in the bed, should you so desire. You can either teach them your tricks (what's hotter than communication?), or you can work your skills while they watch, or otherwise participate—hand over your sex toy of choice. Whatever works! But first, it's time to get busy—alone. If you're already masturbating—and chances are you might be, because five out of ten adult women do—take this as inspiration to do it even more. Beyond feeling great, masturbating is actually good for you, both mentally and physically.

There's bona fide scientific data to back up that it relieves stress, among other fab benefits. And all that with zero health risk! It's kind of like a wonder wellness boost you should add to your life as much as you want to. It's certainly more enjoyable and relaxing than green juice! (No offense to green juice.)

And while you're at it, try chatting with your friends about it. You might learn a thing or two.

THE FIRST TIME

Talk to anyone with a young kid and they will tell you just how natural it is for humans to touch themselves—girls and boys—from a very young age. Kids know what feels good and are innocently free from the kind of knowledge that leads to unnecessary guilt and shame. So they poke and prod their bodies. Some kids even rub on things—toys in the tub or stuffed animals. Menfolk by and large have a comfortable relationship with masturbation and feel at ease playing with themselves. Women, less so. Anecdotally, there are basically two camps of female masturbators, beyond those very early years, when playing with yourself is just exploration, and sexual fantasy is clearly not a part of it. There are the ones who start with purpose and intention around puberty and never stop. And then there are the people who never thought to, or were told not to, or didn't really have the urge to, or wanted to but couldn't figure out how to start.

Members of the latter camp may find themselves being touched by partners or even having penetrative sex *before* they've ever touched themselves. And, for the most part, that's a big sexual disadvantage. When and if you haven't spent the time to figure out what feels good when you're alone, it's probably not the easiest thing to discover with someone else doing it for you. This is obviously a massive generalization, but usually there's some kernel(s) of truth in these sorts of generalizations. Female orgasm with a partner is (generally) easier to achieve when you've already mastered it alone. And (generally), there are less obstacles on the path to pleasure when you know what you like already and can communicate that to a partner (lick this way, fast or slow, no fingers, two fingers, please pass the vibrator, pressure right *here*). There's absolutely nothing wrong with having sex if you have never given yourself a full-fledged orgasm, but you might get there more easily if you know yourself, intimately. There's a reason 47 percent of women had their first orgasm while masturbating; it only takes one special person to get the job done. And that's you.

If, for whatever reason, you find yourself at the end of college or signing your first lease or celebrating your thirty-fifth birthday and you still haven't put your own hand down your own pants, you're not alone. And you may feel a little stuck. Like, really, how *do* you start? Mainly you have to get out of your own head and just go for it. There's no need to get in a sexy mood, or take a bath to relax, unless that's your thing. (On second thought, maybe you do want to get in the bath, especially if you have a handheld showerhead. Water pressure can work wonders.) You don't need to dim the lights and pour yourself a glass of wine, unless you want to. You don't need to shave or decide what to wear, or not wear as the case may be. You don't have to be horny or crushing on yourself to do you. It's not like you've been on a date with yourself all night and the feeling has been building up. Though, if you're super stressed, maybe *that* feeling is built up and can be released—by you. Need a warm-up? Read some erotica, watch some Nancy Meyers, whatever works! For women, the brain is a highly erotic organ; some call it the focal point of female sexuality.

The point is to just *start*. Like, right now.

Still not sure what to do? A few pointers: build up slowly. Don't jump straight in with an unlubricated dildo. That's not fun for anyone, and it won't turn you into a repeat customer. A natural moment to try is at bedtime, or first thing in the morning. But you don't even have to be home in bed. That's one of the big benefits of being a woman—masturbation for the ladies is a fairly self-contained experience. So slide your hand down south and see what works. Gentle or rough. And please do touch *every* part of your vulva. If most women don't come from vaginal penetration alone, it stands to reason that self-love isn't only going to involve fingering. Some women forgo fingers altogether and just concentrate on the clitoris. Don't neglect your breasts or your ass. Both areas can be sensitive. Basically, try it all. And then do it again and again and again. Hit on something that works? Mix it up and try something else.

One other thought—sometimes the first time isn't actually the first time. As in: maybe you masturbate but you've never done it when you have your period—try that as a first. It can help with cramps! Or maybe you haven't masturbated since a nonconsensual experience. Or maybe you've never masturbated while taking antidepressants. If you're newly on an SSRI and it's helping you overall but messing with your libido, masturbation is your friend, maybe even your BFF. Ditto if your hormones are changing—with age, with pregnancy, or post-pregnancy. All those times are masturbation firsts, too. What better way to figure out and explore your sensitivities as your body shifts than in private? Every day you touch yourself is going to be different—a first—and there are always lessons to be learned about your own body.

And if you're truly feeling nothing—no urge, no tension, no arousal—check in with your gyno. Often, if a patient comes in complaining of lack of orgasm with partners, doctors will ask if you're able to achieve it alone. By and large the answer is yes. If you're not feeling it even when you're solo, you could have some hormonal imbalances your doctor can help with. Or you might want to check in with a therapist.

TOYS

If you have a vibrator stashed away in a drawer and haven't used it yet, please put this book down and come back when you have. If you have used one and it was eh, or you've never used one and are in the market, here's some insight into the wonderful world of toys. There is literally something for everyone available right now, thanks, in part, to a whole slew of young female vibrator designers, like the women at Dame Products, who get it and are able to craft from experience.

Now let's be clear, toys aren't a must. Still, some women say their own hands don't cut it; that is, they can't achieve the level of pleasure they want with manual pressure alone. And so a (good) toy can be a gateway to pleasure. And for others who like their hands just fine but who want a bit of spice in their alone sessions: toy time.

To get a toy, you have to shop—online or in person. Shopping IRL is the best way to get a sense of what's available and what materials feel good to touch, and to really understand what these things can do. You can turn toys on and hear how loud they buzz (a quiet toy is key if you're easily distracted or if you live with roommates!). You can also ask questions, because there are an overwhelming number of vibrators on the market today in all shapes and sizes—bullets and rabbits and wands and wand attachments and so on (and, no, not every toy has to actually look like a penis if that's not what you want). Some women may feel shy or even embarrassed to ask questions about sex toys in person. But really, truly, the salespeople in these shops love to talk about toys and don't judge. They're just there to help you find what's right for you.

A vibrator is an awesome investment, and you surely want to get the best one for you. If you're not up for asking an expert questions face-to-face, do some online research. It's incredible all the things you can read about that maybe you haven't considered, like, some toys are not best for first-timers. Or that it's critical to match the shape of a toy to how you personally like to feel pleasure (inside or outside or both, aka dual-action). If you like to only focus on your clitoris, you'll want one kind of a toy; if you like a more broad, all-over buzz, you'll need a different shape. Do you like variety? Try a multitasking, versatile toy with multiple intensity levels (there are many). Do you want a hands-free experience? For some women to experience orgasm, they need to mindfully let all their muscles relax enough to let them spasm, so having one hand tensely working a toy can disrupt this process. Do you want silicone or stainless steel or even glass? Do you want something battery-operated or is there an electrical outlet right next to your bed?

If you feel overwhelmed, like there is so much more to the world of toys than you realized, just order something basic online and get going. A pro tip from our friend Alexandra Fine, cofounder of Dame Products, which makes some seriously revolutionary sex toys: since most women don't orgasm from penetration alone, you might not want to start out with a penetrative toy unless you already know you're super into it. (If that's all you have, never fear, you can use a vibrating internal toy externally, of course.) But she can't say what, exactly, to buy first because "sex toys are like wine"; only you know what's great for you. It's never one size fits all. Focus on vibration, texture, size, and if it's insertable. Once you've had one toy experience, it can inform your future shopping. It's always OK to upgrade later on, when you know better what you're specifically interested in seeking—maybe it's something to help you try anal or to find your G-spot (see page 204), whatever interests you.

When you're done with your toy selection(s), don't forget about lubricant. Yeah, you might have enough natural lubrication, but lube is great stuff. The more the merrier, and it will make the whole process more comfortable no matter what, so why not? You definitely want one made with organic ingredients and without harsh synthetics that can hurt rather than help your vagina (for more on the wonder that is lube, check out page 220). And avoid silicone lubricant, as it can actually break down the silicone in most toys—kind of like how the only thing that can hurt a diamond is a diamond. Oils can work, too, but not if you're also using a condom on your toy; oil can break down condoms. A water-based lube will be good for use with all toy materials—and you.

Finally, do your vagina a favor: keep all toys clean! Some materials, like silicone, are said to be easier to clean than others. Follow manufacturer instructions, especially for battery-operated or electrical toys. Usually all you need is mild soap and warm water. Not up for getting out of bed to lather your toy when you're feeling lazy post-sesh? Keep some wipes by the bed

MATERIAL WORLD

There are no real regulations around adult toys, which is unhappy news for vaginas. Manufacturers basically need only to prove they're making safe electronics. So it's up to you to be smart when shopping to find the safest toys. They come in so many different materials—plastic, obviously, but there are also glass and stainless steel and even wood ones. Most of these materials aren't tested for safety for the way they are going to be used, though glass is inert and stainless steel is generally considered safe. For wood, you'd want to know what was used to seal it to make it nonporous. But since the majority of toys are plastic, it's worth spending a few minutes to find out what kind of plastic is being used. Just be smart about it: don't be in a huge rush, ask questions, do your research. It's the rare sex toy with a materials label so this information can be maddeningly tricky to come by.

Why bother? Not all plastic is what's called body-safe—and be aware when shopping that even that term *body-safe* is unregulated! And you're putting this in and around your *vagina*—a super porous and precious part of your body. You want that plastic to be safe.

Take PVC/vinyl. To make it soft and flexible, it usually contains hormone-disrupting chemicals. These can release into the air you breathe and break down when in contact with heat and maybe even bodily fluid. Avoid it. If you can't figure out what's PVC by reading labels, a good rule of thumb is to avoid "jelly" plastic toys or anything that has that unmistakable new plastic smell, you know, that kind that wafts out of new cars or from sneakers or new shower curtains. Also bad: jelly toys are porous, can't be sterilized, and can "melt" into other plastics if stored touching them between sessions. Using jelly plastic with certain kinds of personal lubricant may even help its chemical components migrate out of the plastic and into your body. If you already own and like your jelly toy, it's a good idea to consider using a condom on it to protect your vagina.

Here's some good news for women who love their flexible plastic toys: a lot of these aren't jelly plastic; they're made of silicone, which is considered by and large safe for sex toys. You do want to make sure it is 100 percent medical-grade silicone and not part silicone and part some other random and unidentifiable filler material. When a toy is 100 percent silicone, it's said to be nonporous and can be sterilized. A good rule of thumb is that real silicone won't smell like a new shower curtain, and it won't change color, texture, or shape as you bend it. So, on top of everything else you have on your mind when toy shopping, don't neglect to read the small print on packaging to figure out what a gadget is made of. Ask questions if you're not sure what's what. Then you won't have to worry about materials when you're playing—that's not hot.

for a quick clean, and later on you can do a deeper scrub. Just make sure whatever ingredients are in the wipe are something you deem OK to use on your vagina. And whatever you do, don't use harsh detergent; that residue can irritate your vagina. Keep it clean and you'll be good to go. And go and go and go.

HEALTH BENEFITS

The benefits of masturbation, like sex (see chapter six), are no joke fantastic—both mentally as well as physically. What's better than knowing something fabulous is also medically recommended? It's kind of like how red wine has antioxidants: hell yes. The basic deal is orgasms cause your body to release a bunch of hormones, including oxytocin, the "love" hormone. These reduce all kinds of bad-for-you things in your body, including lowering cortisol, a notorious stress hormone, which has been linked to weight-loss issues, inflammation, stress eating, insomnia . . . you name it, cortisol seems to be to blame. But give yourself an orgasm to combat that cortisol and then you're more than chill, you're healthier. Here are some of the many ways masturbation can benefit your health.

Relieve tension.

A little sexual tension can be, well, sexy. But tension overall isn't good for you, especially if there is no way to get rid of it.

It's heart-healthy.

Orgasms have been linked to lower blood pressure and lower risk of heart disease. Masturbation probably won't beneficially raise your heart rate as much as going for a run or even an energetic romp with a partner, but both help your heart. Win-win.

You're getting sleepy. . . .

There are plenty of people who pop off to sleep, literally, using masturbation like natural Ambien. Awake and stressed at night? Do you, then get back to sleep. After orgasm, a hormone called prolactin is released, which makes you tired. Even if you're not headed directly to ZZZs, prolactin is proven to trigger relaxation.

Privacy can be revealing.

According to the Center for Sexual Health, only 64 percent of women reported having had an orgasm at their last sexual encounter. When you're alone, you're in charge of upping that statistic. Also, according to the Kinsey Institute, up to 70 percent of women need clitoral stimulation to orgasm. Again, when you're alone, this is much easier to attend to. It bears repeating when you're comfortable with and feeling confident about your body and how it functions, this can translate well to when you're with a partner.

Boost your immune system.

Research has shown that people who orgasm regularly take less sick days. This is precisely why masturbation should be considered a critical part of a wellness routine. Speaking of work, studies even show that a "wank break" (instead of a smoke break) at work can increase your focus. Not that we're encouraging you to get it on with yourself in the communal bathrooms, but, still, good to know.

Reduce pain.

Got cramps? Try masturbating. There are hormones orgasm releases that basically raise your pain threshold. This means it can help more than cramps. Give it a whirl for a headache. Studies have shown that stimulation—even without orgasm—can help block both back and leg pain.

Boost libido!

Research shows playing with yourself raises the capacity for more orgasms thanks to increased vaginal lubrication and blood flow. Depending on what toys you use, if any, you may also be boosting elasticity. But sexuality is more than physical; it's also mental. The more you masturbate, the more you think about sex (even solo sex), the more you're going to want it. All of this makes the experience better—alone or with a partner.

Get fit.

Orgasm can strengthen your muscle tone—in both the pelvic and anal areas. It also makes you mentally fit, as in it can increase your self-esteem and up your body image. Feeling toned and hot, in turn, make you more interested in sex.

It's risk-free.

There is nothing not to love about unlimited pleasure with zero risk of STIs or pregnancy. Bring it on.

THREE QUESTIONS

1 I'M INTERESTED IN PORN, BUT I'M ON THE FENCE. I HAVE A FRIEND WHO SAYS IT'S HORRIBLE TO WATCH BECAUSE NOT ALL SEX WORKERS ARE TREATED WELL. AND YET, I LIKE TO MASTURBATE WHILE WATCHING. IS THAT BAD?

First off, there are (basically) no bads, especially when it comes to masturbation. Also, you're not alone in what you like to do alone. There are a lot of people who enjoy porn while they masturbate, including women. Pornhub.com's Dr. Laurie Betito says about 35 percent of their users are women. As long as you're not hurting anyone or yourself, everything is on the table. There should be no guilt. But what feels enticing isn't always politically correct. And so there are people, like your friend, who avoid porn because they don't feel it can be empowering, or that it objectifies women, or supports sex slavery. Actually, it objectifies sex—not just women or men—reducing it to body parts and stripping it of key elements of great sex, like connection. It's staged, a show, not real! Porn allows us to get off through fantasy—maybe even about something you aren't into when it comes to partners, but you like to think about when you're alone. Maybe it will help you to know there are actually sex-positive pro-porn feminists out there advocating for the rights of sex workers who like porn. The going argument there is that acknowledging the role of fantasy, including porn, in arousal sheds both shame and taboo. And, really, we shouldn't be expected to have 100 percent PC fantasies. They invite an honest discussion about women's bodies (as well as consent and safer sex). If you're torn, do some research. It's a lively debate. And, while you're at it, check out what's commonly referred to as "female-friendly" porn if you haven't yet. There are many more natural options, like real (not fake) breasts, foreplay, un- or less-waxed women, consent, plus women and couples who look like they might actually be enjoying themselves, not acting. There are even feminist porn awards! Whatever you could consider empowering, it's out there. 24/7 streaming free accessibility has for sure given way to some pretty extreme and graphic gonzo porn, but that's not all that's available. If you want to watch porn, there are more thoughtful ways to stream it. Another option for a good visual is to set up a mirror and watch yourself. Or if you're just in it for the story, pick up a book of erotica or read some online. Then mentally cast your fantasy any way you want to. If you're feeling uncomfortable because something feels hot in the moment but later, intellectually, it makes you uncomfortable, don't be so hard on yourself. Fantasy is just fantasy. Don't read so much into it if you fantasizo about sex stuff you wouldn't actually do IRL. You're not bad if you think about new things as you masturbate. Give yourself permission to explore.

2 I HAVE A BOYFRIEND, BUT I STILL LIKE TO MASTURBATE. AM I CHEATING ON HIM? HE SEEMS TO THINK SO, LIKE I SHOULD BE SAVING THAT FOR HIM.

Do not even for one second think of masturbating as cheating or that you're supposed to be "saving" your pleasure for your partner. Puh-lease. This is your alone time. And no doubt your partner is having some alone time, too. Does that bother you? The more you orgasm, the easier it is for you to orgasm. That's science worth repeating. If for some reason your partner is jealous of your masturbating, ask him or her why. Sounds like an honest conversation is in order. You could also ask him to join you, but only if you want. Lots of people find that hot.

3 CAN YOU GET ADDICTED TO MASTURBATING?

No, no, no, no, and no. Got it? You cannot get addicted to masturbating. Not even a little bit. And you cannot get addicted to a vibrator, either. The worst you can do is make yourself a little sore or maybe a little numb. One caveat here: if you're asking because you're missing work meetings and, say, your sister's birthday party, because you're at home doing you, it's probably time to have a little chat with your therapist or another medical professional who knows you best.

CHAPTER 4

HOW TO NOT MAKE BABIES:

ALL THE BIRTH CONTROL OPTIONS

Whether you're out there having a blast meeting new partners or enjoying the partner you currently have (over and over again), there's a little something you might be trying to avoid: getting pregnant. Most of us spend forty or more years in our reproductive phase of life, so this simple act preoccupies some women for a big chunk of time. Avoiding pregnancy is a necessary part of a healthy heterosexual sex life, since making babies is exactly what our amazing female reproductive systems are designed to do. There are a whole bunch of ways to block egg and sperm from ever meeting (or from implanting if they do meet). And yet the unintended pregnancy rate in the United States hovers at about 45 percent (higher than any other developed country). Guess what? This isn't because all those women aren't using contraception. It's because some birth control has higher efficacy rates than others. And it's because of human error; not all of us use contraception correctly—you know, like missing taking your pill. Only about 14 percent of women who do not use contraception at all were responsible for approximately 50 percent of those unintended pregnancies. The highest pregnancy rates, not surprisingly, occur among young women aged twenty to twenty-four, and those who are socio-economically disadvantaged. Accessing birth control is an issue for more than twenty million women in the United States, and data shows that certain racial/ethnic groups also have higher rates of unintended pregnancies.

The impacts of unintended pregnancies can be traumatic. They can throw lives off indefinitely, affecting education, finances, mental health, and so much more. But they don't have to happen if you have access to and can afford birth control; there are so many different contraceptive options out there, including some super long-acting ones that prevent pregnancy more than 99 percent of the time. There's everything from male or female sterilization (not an option if you do want to have kids one day) to implants to IUDs. These require no compliance from you—you don't have to remember to take that pill, or insert a ring, or put in a sponge. You're always covered. So why aren't more women choosing these methods? Access is an issue. Education is an issue. Insurance is an issue. Cost is an issue. And even when you have insurance, access, and cash, birth control can be a tale of compromises. Many women love what they're using, but generally there's no one-size-fits-all. You can lament that the options suck because of, well, patriarchy, but think about it. When you're trying to thwart nature and keep your body from doing what it's built to do, of course there isn't always a perfect answer. It's all about educating yourself about your options and making the right decision for you.

Some contraception feels so right, so effortless in your body, that you won't even notice it—that's the goal. But with others, you might spot, you might get headaches or mood changes or cramps. Or you might have to stop in the very middle of just the right kind of do-me-now heat and take a pause to go insert something and maybe spermicide will drip out of you. Here's the thing, even if your method is not totally perfect, it's still awesome. As in: birth control is literally about controlling when you want to give birth, to bring a child into this world. That's freedom—a freedom women have not historically enjoyed and which many women around the world still don't. Get on top of that, take charge of your reproductive health, and find the contraceptive method that works best for your unique body.

Finding your best birth control may take a moment; be patient. If you don't adore what you're currently using, take the time to research other methods and make a change. Planned Parenthood, Bedsider, Centers for Disease Control and Prevention, the World Health Organization, and many other organizations are solid resources. Some of their websites even let you take a quiz or personalize your search to determine what options will match your specific needs. Then consult with your doctor about your research; you may read about something cool-sounding you're sure is just the thing for you, but your doc—be it your gyno, GP, pediatrician, midwife, or nurse practitioner—can advise on how your health history and your family health history may determine what's medically best. If you're trying something new and don't like it, keep changing until you find a method you're comfortable with. If something was working well with one partner and not so much with a new partner, mix things up. Just make sure to use backup methods as you make changes, in case you're uncovered as you transition from one type of birth control to another.

THE MIGHTY CONDOM

Speaking of backup methods: YOU HAVE TO USE CONDOMS. Like *seriously*. Before we even get into what kinds of birth control are out there it must be said loud and clear that being on birth control does not at all get you out of using condoms. So we're saying it. It doesn't matter what other birth control method you are using. Condoms are the only contraceptive available that protects our bodies from STIs, which can last (or even shorten) a lifetime. To repeat: no other method of contraception can safeguard your body from sexually transmitted diseases and infections, including HIV/AIDS. So they

THE FEMALE CONDOM: A RARITY

The next time you're hanging out with a group of friends, take an informal poll: Who here has used a female condom? Chances are the answer will be no one. Female condoms are such a fantastic women-in-charge idea. But they just haven't taken off. If you're interested in using them, give them a trial run or two without your partner first; they can be a bit tricky to put in, which means they have a fairly high failure rate of 21 percent—as in twenty-one out of one hundred people using them as their main method of birth control will get pregnant each year. Though if you use them perfectly every single time, Planned Parenthood says their effectiveness is 95 percent; practice makes not entirely perfect. Basically it's two rings with a loose condom barrier in between. You insert the upper ring around your cervix, sort of like you would with a diaphragm. The second ring hangs just outside your vagina. A cool thing is they can be inserted hours before having sex—check the product packaging for exact timing. And you can use them when you're having your period. When the moment arises, you guide your partner through the second ring and into your vagina, making sure the penis is actually in the condom and not on either side of it, entering you unsheathed. When you're done doing your thing, removal takes some getting used to. After your partner pulls out, you twist the condom at the exterior ring to trap the ejaculate, then unhook the interior ring, and discard. They're not expensive and are available over-the-counter, but most stores that sell male condoms don't carry them. They're just not popular enough—yet.

always have to be part of the deal. (For more information on STIs and condoms, check out chapter five.) Since the condoms most commonly used go on penises and require male participation, some women think it's not their job to carry them in their purse or store them in their bedside table. Don't be that person. Be the woman carrying condoms at all times, because sex is awesome and being safe shows you give a damn about your health. Stash them in your wallet, your car, your gym bag. Load them into the drawer next to your bed, your medicine cabinet, your office. Get good at rolling them on. And require them: Every. Single. Time. You. Have. Penetrative. Sex. Please and thank you.

Condoms also pair beautifully with all other birth control methods and increase contraceptive efficacy with minimal to no side effects. Sensitive to latex? No problem, try a nonlatex condom. Condoms are also widely accessible, don't require a visit to your doctor, and don't cost a lot (some clinics and schools even offer them for free). No STI is worth a condom's supposed disadvantages. People can complain all they want about decreased sensitivity, erection issues, lack of intimacy, or reduction in spontaneity in the moment, but any of those concerns is nothing compared to, say, undetected chlamydia that leads to pelvic inflammatory disease that leads to infertility before you've even had a moment to consider your fertility. There's nothing more intimate about unprotected sex that results in an

STI. How about herpes that will mean, years later, you may not be able to have the vaginal childbirth you want? Pass the condoms, please! If you have a partner resistant to condoms, swipe left. There are so many other people out there who are more than happy to roll one on to get in your pants. They should be equally interested in safeguarding their own health. Hook up with and date those guys. And work with them to find a condom that's the right material, fit, and thinness for both of you.

Here are a few other things to know about condoms: Latex can break down if paired with oil-based lubricants (that means mineral oils like baby oil as well as petroleum jelly). So don't use those as lubes. Also, men are not supposed to wear more than one. Double bagging sounds super protected but actually it causes friction that can lead to rips or tears in the condoms. And while condoms are great to buddy up with other birth control methods, you don't want to use a male condom with a female condom; that can also cause them to break. Other things that can weaken condoms include vaginal estrogen and oil-based antifungal creams (like what you use when you have a yeast infection, see page 35). If you're ever in doubt, ask your doctor or your pharmacist if a cream or a lubricant is OK to use with condoms.

PERFECTING THE ART OF THE CONDOM

The typical use efficacy rate of male condoms is 82 percent, while perfect use is 98 percent! The considerable difference between typical and perfect use comes down to human error, not failure of the product. Condoms are classified and strictly regulated by the FDA as a class II medical device to provide, among other things, assurance about effectiveness. That means one brand works just as well as another. It's your job to know how to use them perfectly. Here's how.

START FRESH. Use a new condom every single time you have vaginal, oral, or anal sex. Condoms are not meant to be reused.

MAKE SURE IT'S ON THE *ENTIRE* TIME. Guess what? Starting sexual activity without a condom and then putting it on midway through is *not* foreplay. It's a bad idea. Skin-to-skin genital contact is risky behavior! Wear that condom start to finish.

CARE FOR YOUR CONDOMS. Check out your condom's expiration date; vintage, in this case, is no good. Inspect the package, too; it should be sealed and not damaged. Store condoms in a cool, dry place. Don't keep them in a hot spot for long periods of time. If your partner has one tucked in a wallet he keeps endlessly in his back pocket, grab another.

OPEN GENTLY. Don't use scissors or teeth to open a condom. Go slow, even if you're feeling rushed.

PUT IT ON CORRECTLY. Place the unwrapped condom on the head of the penis, making sure the rim is on the outside so you can unroll it down the shaft. Pinch the end of the condom to remove air from the receptacle tip and unroll the condom all the way down the shaft to the base of the penis. That's it. (If your partner is uncircumcised, have him show you his preferred and most comfortable foreskin placement, then unroll.) Confused? Watch a video!

LUBE, GLORIOUS LUBE. Who doesn't love lube? Use only water-based or silicone-based lubricants with condoms; oil-based lubes can weaken the latex.

BUDDY UP. Use another form of birth control with your condom if you want some backup. But do not use two condoms; the friction can cause breakage.

BACK OUT! Shoo your partner out of you as soon as you're all done. Some men lose their erections very quickly post ejaculation and accidents can happen as the condom becomes loose on a less than totally hard penis. Semen can get out where you do not want it.

HOLD THE RIM. Either you or your partner needs to hold on to the base of the condom as he pulls out to avoid slippage or spillage. Then make sure the used condom is carefully removed from your vaginal vicinity and tossed into the garbage, not flushed down the toilet. They could clog your pipes and might reemerge in your bathroom at an inconvenient moment, or they'll wind up in public waterways intact; unlike other flushable waste, condoms are not biodegradable.

MAKING THE CHOICE

Now that you're a condom pro, it's time to consider pairing those condoms with your own birth control, if you want. There's nothing more powerful than a woman accessing birth control in any form. How to choose? There is no one-size-fits-all option.

- First, you need it to be effective. Makes sense, but not all methods are created equal. There's a reason doctors are currently gung ho about LARCs (long-acting reversible contraception) that are more than 99 percent effective, like the IUD and the implant: they're responsible for a significant decrease in teen pregnancy rates. The majority of LARC methods are hormonal, minus the copper IUD. If you don't want anything containing hormones, that will lead you down another path.

- Second, you need to make sure whatever you opt for is something that makes sense for you to use. If you're not someone who is good at remembering to take medicine, don't go on the pill. The ring or the patch might be a better fit.

- Third, you want something that makes your body feel, well, like your body. The shot might make you gain weight, the pill might make you extra moody, the hormonal IUD might make you spot, or a copper one could make you bleed more heavily during your period. Don't freak out in advance about side effects you read about or that your best friend might have. Our adviser Dr. Angela, ob-gyn, points out that different women react differently to a given method. You may have a totally unique reaction to the ring compared to your very own sister. You just won't know how your body responds until you try something. And, keep in mind, if you have a side effect you don't like, there's always another way to go.

As you weigh your options and try to narrow them down to one choice, there are a bunch of other things to consider. Like your long-term plans—if you do want to get pregnant sometime in the near future, choose something that's super reversible. It takes women a while to return to fertility with the shot, so that wouldn't be right for someone eager to get pregnant soon. And, of course, there is price to consider, especially if you don't have insurance or your insurance won't cover birth control or certain kinds of birth control—fully or at all. IUDs are expensive up front but can be inside you for three to ten years, depending on which kind you choose, so the price evens out over time and is often cheaper than most other methods in the long run. But if you want it taken out in a year to try to get pregnant, an IUD wouldn't make financial sense.

You'll also need to talk to your doctor about your health; some conditions, diseases, and even breastfeeding can contraindicate certain birth control methods. Breast cancer patients, for

THE TALK

Whether you're going on birth control for the first time or you're changing your current method, you're going to want to talk to your doctor. Try not to go to that appointment convinced you're absolutely going on one specific method. Be open to other possibilities. The conversation, ideally, should not be rushed. Your doctor should listen carefully to your history, plus your current needs and desires. Your doctor should ask if you want to get your period every month and listen to what side effects would be tolerable to you. And they should share with you information on all the methods available–from sterilization to hormonal to nonhormonal options. When someone comes to her office to talk about birth control, Dr. Angela considers it her responsibility to present *everything* that is out there. Her goal is to give women enough information so they can make an informed decision. She offers pros and cons. And she always tells patients–of all ages–to use condoms. In other words, she's the shit. If your doctor is rushing you or refusing to offer information on, say, fertility awareness method or anything they deem not effective enough, go make an appointment with another doctor. It's up to you.

example, might need to use something nonhormonal, depending on their receptor status. People who have migraines might also need specific kinds of birth control. If you're obese, some methods are more effective than others. So schedule an appointment and go have a good long, open, and honest chat with your ob-gyn that spans every option currently available to you, from LARCs to emergency birth control. Of course there's always abstinence. But doesn't it feel like a shame to give up sex entirely just to avoid pregnancy? There are risks and side effects from everything we do all day long, but we still get out of bed and go out in the world. Besides, data shows there's even a pregnancy risk from "abstinence," so either people don't understand the definition of that word or they can't resist the urge. We get it. In case you're wondering, the chance of getting pregnant if you're using absolutely nothing is 85 percent in one year if you're sexually active. So choose something effective, use it correctly, and enjoy yourself.

Here are some questions to think about and ask as you weigh all the pros and cons of what's currently on the market.

- How long does it take for your chosen method to be effective?

- How does this method actually work to keep you from getting pregnant? What's the mechanism—does it inhibit ovulation, change your cervical mucus, thin your uterine lining?

- What are the common side effects of any given method? Nausea? Weight gain? You want to know.
- Why would someone not be able to use a certain kind of birth control?
- Does the method put you at higher risk for any diseases? If so, how and which ones?
- Does data show the method protects against any cancers or, say, pelvic inflammatory disease? If so, how?
- How long does it take to return to fertility once you go off this method?
- How long can you be on this method safely?
- Are there any contraindications?
- If you have an STI, is this method safe for you?
- What will this method do to your period: Will it make you spot, bleed more, bleed less? Will it help with cramps or make them worse? Will it help with acne or make it worse? Will it make your breasts more or less sore?
- What will this method do to your cervical mucus?
- Will it take a few months for your body to get used to it—what should you expect?

- If you miss taking or inserting your method, do you need a backup method?
- Will this method decrease bone density?
- Do you need a vaginal exam before starting your method? A Pap?
- Do you need STI testing or a pregnancy test before starting a method?
- Can you go on your new method on the same day you go off your old method? If you switch methods, how long should you use backup protection?
- Can a partner see or feel this method?

THE BIRTH CONTROL MENU

Here's a little bit of useful info on every birth control option currently available to you—more than you might get from a pamphlet you'd skim in a doctor's waiting room, but not a true deep dive. As you get closer to finding the method you know you want to use, definitely do your own research. You should know all there is to know about what you're inserting in, wearing on, or swallowing into your unique body.

COMPARE AND CONTRAST

Power to Decide, the campaign to prevent unplanned pregnancy, created an amazing must-read chart of all birth control options for their website, Bedsider.org. It's a nonprofit, which means it's not funded by the companies that make birth control, or our government. The site also includes efficacy ratings for each option, which we've included in the following pages so you're completely in the know.

	IUD	THE IMPLANT	THE SHOT	THE RING	THE PATCH	THE PILL	CONDOM
EFFECTIVENESS	★	★	●	●	●	●	◐
SIDE EFFECTS	●	●	●	●	●	●	★
STI PREVENTION	✕	✕	✕	✕	✕	✕	★
EASY TO HIDE	★	★	★	●	●	●	◐
DO ME NOW Some folks say the ability to be spontaneous (with nothing to worry about in the moment) can make sex better.	★	★	★	★	★	★	◐
PARTY READY Party-ready methods are taken care of long before you head out for the night, but need to be combined with a condom to prevent STIs.	★	★	★	★	★	●	◐

MOST EFFECTIVE

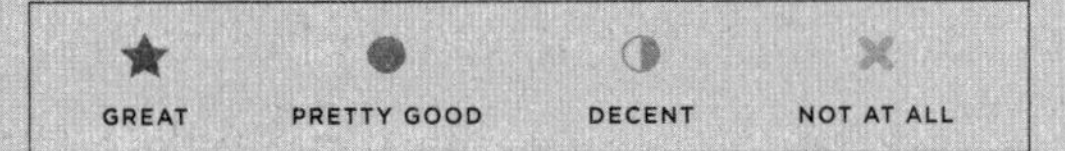

– Sterilization –

Perfect use: greater than 99 percent

Typical use: greater than 99 percent†

If you are totally 100 percent sure you and your partner do not ever want to have biological kids—*ever*—then getting your tubes tied or your partner having a vasectomy is a highly effective and hormone-free way to prevent pregnancy. It can take a while to come to this conclusion, so sterilization tends mainly to be an option for people who have already had some kids and would prefer not to have more. It's also a good option for women for whom getting pregnant presents a big health risk. The procedure (male or female) isn't cheap. Of course, once you're sterilized, you never have to shell out money for birth control again (other than condoms to protect from STIs, depending on who you're sleeping with). It can be emotionally difficult to decide which partner is getting snipped, and there are various methods to choose from. If you're interested in sterilization, do some research and make an appointment to talk through all the options and possible side effects with your doctor.

– Abstinence –

100% effective but *only* if you really, truly don't have sex

Not having sex works well for not getting pregnant. But then again you won't be having vaginal sex. Which can be a big

† The perfect use and typical use ratings on the following pages come from Bedsider.org.

bummer. If it's not an issue for you to give up, go for it. There are certainly plenty of other ways to get off with committed partners and new-to-you partners alike. Keep in mind putting a penis inside you—unsheathed—for just a little bit but not for the whole time is neither abstinence nor a good idea. You could still get pregnant and you could also contract an STI. If you're going to be abstinent, you have to embrace it and communicate it clearly to all partners. It's not a bad idea to keep a condom on you or even be on a backup method in case you change your mind.

BARRIER METHODS

Don't want extra hormones in your body? You're not alone. Some women worry about the long-term effects of taking hormones, despite plenty of data available on its safety. Others find they feel "crazy" or have no sex drive or don't quite feel like themselves on hormones. Barrier methods—which include cervical caps, diaphragms, and sponges—are going to be for you. Unfortunately they are not the most effective birth control methods on the market, but if you use condoms at the same time, as you should be if you're not in a committed monogamous relationship where both partners have been tested, that can increase efficacy rates. Barrier methods tend to involve getting your hands all up inside yourself. So do it!

– Diaphragm –

Perfect use: 94 percent

Typical use: 88 percent

These are barriers, typically made from silicone, that are used with spermicide. They come in several sizes—you get fitted at an appointment with your doctor. There's also a one-size-fits-most version that does not technically require a fitting, but does require a prescription. You might want to do a test run at your doctor's office anyway, just to make sure it's comfortable and you can insert and remove it without issue. For the multisized kind, you need to be refitted if you gain or lose a considerable amount of weight or if you have a child. They can for sure take some getting used to. You fill it with spermicide (a deal breaker if you're allergic to spermicide) and insert (with clean hands) within two hours before you know you're going to have sex. If you put it in before that two-hour window, like up to three to six hours before sex, that's OK, too, but you'd need to reinsert spermicide. If you wind up having a few rounds of sex, you'll also need to insert additional spermicide in your vagina (do not remove the diaphragm!), which can get things pretty lubed up. Then, after all is said and done, you leave it in place for another six hours. Next, you have to remove it (you unhook it with your finger and try not to spill the body-temperature spermicide it's holding as you slide it out), wash it, and store it. You can't leave it in for more than twenty-four hours because it elevates the risk of toxic shock syndrome (see page 79). If you're using lubricant with a diaphragm, it has to be water- or silicone-based. Oil-based lube can break down the silicone. Some women are sensitive to the spermicide even if they're not fully allergic to it. It can change vaginal pH and create irritation. Diaphragms can also increase risk for urinary tract infections. Some men claim they can feel them inside their partners, but thankfully if you put it in correctly you yourself won't feel it. It can also be knocked out of place by very energetic sex. The good news is that it's effective immediately after you insert it. Once you get used to the routine, using a diaphragm and knowing how to check it for leaks becomes, well, routine.

– Cervical Cap –

Perfect use: not available

Typical use: 71 to 86 percent

Caps are quite similar to diaphragms in terms of insertion, removal, and care. Again, there are several sizes of caps and you'll need to get fitted by your doctor. Some health clinics will have them in stock, but not all drugstores do, so you might need to mail order one once you have your prescription. You can have the same cap, if it doesn't have a hole, for several years. The difference between caps and diaphragms is that caps are a lot smaller and their efficacy rate stinks, especially for women who have already had children. You're definitely going to want a backup method with a cap. Like a diaphragm, you fill it with spermicide and insert it up to six hours prior to having sex, have to reinsert more spermicide if you're going for several rounds of fun, and then leave it in for at least six hours before removing it. The spermicide can interfere with vaginal pH, which in turn can cause irritation. Caps aren't a great option unless you're in a relationship where getting pregnant wouldn't be a hardship. While partners don't usually complain of being able to feel caps, it could technically get thrust out of position if things are really raucous or by a particularly large penis. Some women report an increase in UTIs when using cervical caps.

– Sponge –

Perfect use: 80 to 91 percent

Typical use: 76 to 88 percent

A sponge is literally a small sponge, typically made of polyurethane, which contains spermicide. You use a small amount of water, like two to three tablespoons, to activate the spermicide before insertion, then you insert it kind of like you would a tampon (with clean hands) when you know you're going to have sex. If you're out and about, you'll have to remember to take one with you. One dimpled side fits over the cervix, and there's a loop on the other side to help you pull it out. You'll need to follow the exact directions on the product packaging, but usually a sponge is effective for up to twenty-four hours and can be used for more than one round of sex during that time. It has to be left in place for around six hours once you're done. You don't want to leave it in for more than thirty hours. Spermicide allergy or sensitivity are an issue with sponges, as they are for a cap or a diaphragm. The efficacy rate isn't great, but it's better for women who have not had a child yet. They are sold in drugstores with no prescription, so no doctor visit is needed to use sponges.

INTRAUTERINE DEVICE (IUD)

It's a fairly incredible thing that you can go to your doctor, have an IUD—basically a T-shaped piece of plastic either embedded with hormones or coiled in copper—inserted in your uterus, and pretty much not have to worry about pregnancy for between three to ten years, depending on which model you have. And you literally don't need to do anything: no pills to take, no patches to remember, no spermicide to put in a cap. That's freedom. If you don't want a hormonal IUD, you can have a copper one. IUDs, like any method of birth control, have pros and cons. But they really will keep you protected—just not from STIs. Outside the United States, the IUD is the most popular method of birth control. If you're ever feeling concerned because it just feels too convenient to be true, you can pop a (clean!) finger inside you and feel its strings for reassurance it's there. They don't hang down like a tampon outside of your vagina; they're internal. And you're never supposed to pull or tug on them. Your doctor can check them at your yearly checkup, too. (And yes you can—carefully—use tampons and even menstrual cups when you have an IUD—Planned Parenthood refers to them as next-door neighbors. One is in your uterus, the other in your vagina.) If you think you feel the actual IUD with your finger, you can always have it looked at and adjusted by your doctor. Other than that, if your body takes to it well, you won't know it is there. (And neither will your partner, especially as those strings soften over time.) There are a few medical conditions that don't work with IUDs, so that's a conversation you'll have with your doctor before choosing one. You'll also want to discuss the various risks of IUDs, like uterine perforation, or what to do if it falls out. For a while IUDs were used mainly for women who already had children, but now the medical community agrees they can absolutely be used in women who have not yet had a baby. They can be expensive, depending on your insurance coverage, though the fee up front evens out over time, considering how long they last. Keep in mind that the way medical billing works these days, there will be a charge for the device and another charge for the doctor who does the insertion. Some health clinics offer services on a sliding scale, so ask questions if you're concerned about cost.

Speaking of insertion, some people say it hurts like hell when an IUD goes in your uterus. Others are less sensitive. There may be some brief cramping after insertion. Many women report spotting for up to several months between periods. If this is unbearable, or even just uncomfortable, you can always have your IUD removed. When either kind of IUD is removed, there's a rapid return of fertility—key for women who become interested in getting pregnant. When it comes time to take it out, call your doctor for advice. IUD removal is usually the kind of thing you want a medical professional to do, but there are some studies that show women can take them out on their own without an issue.

– Hormonal IUD –

Perfect use: greater than 99 percent

Typical use: greater than 99 percent

Here's how it works: a small amount of progesterone (well, actually a synthetic version called progestin) is released from the IUD locally in your uterus—not in your entire system, which means detectible levels of progestin in your blood is very, very low. This thins out your uterine lining and thickens cervical mucus to keep sperm from reaching there. Unlike, say, the birth control pill, it does not overtake and redo your own cycle. Many women with a hormonal IUD even ovulate and get their periods, though they get lighter over time—despite increased spotting in the early months. There are a number of hormonal IUDs on the market currently that last up to five years, though at least one brand is in the process of trying to get a seven-year FDA approval.

– Copper IUD –

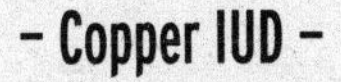

Perfect use: greater than 99 percent

Typical use: greater than 99 percent

Copper inside your uterus prevents sperm and egg from meeting in several ways. It's a potent spermicide because it can literally disable sperm. And it also thickens cervical mucus, making it harder for any undisabled sperm to swim. Even if an egg and a sperm manage to meet, they aren't able to implant because copper creates an inflammatory response in the uterus, creating an inhospitable environment for sperm and egg. Some—but not all—women with a copper IUD report an increase in period flow and sometimes added cramping. Still, it's a highly effective option for women who would like hormone-free birth control. And it can last a decade, or even longer. You won't know how your body reacts until you try it. Concerned about what sperm-killing copper might do in the rest of your system? Data shows the levels are far too low to harm human health.

HORMONAL BIRTH CONTROL

Hormonal birth control is highly effective stuff, though some types are more so than others. Despite the fact that the majority of women using birth control are on a hormonal version, some women don't like the idea of tweaking their hormones. If you're going to go on hormonal birth control, it pays to do your research to even understand what tweaking hormones means. Dig in to learn about the mechanisms of how hormones work to prevent pregnancy, and how synthetic hormones mimic and overtake our own cycles and block ovulation. If hormones concern you, there are some methods that use less, including some that are progesterone-only. Our friend and family-planning goddess Dr. Lauren MacAfee says the patch puts the most hormones into your system, followed by the pill, then the ring. It's also worth digging into what you think hormones might do to your body. These medications all have a substantial amount of long-term safety data—they have to in order to be available to us. They're highly regulated and highly tested. If you're curious about cancer links, check out the American Cancer Society's website, Cancer .org. It maintains a list of which birth controls raise the risk for various cancers, as well as which methods lower risks for other cancers. It's never black-and-white. And then weigh the pros and cons with your own health concerns. Beyond keeping you from getting pregnant, your birth control pill may be saving you from debilitating periods and cramps. That's a big pro. Besides the hormonal IUD, your hormonal birth control options are the patch, the pill, the ring, the shot, and the implant. Read on to find out which one is right for you, listed here in order of efficacy.

– Implant –

Perfect use: greater than 99 percent

Typical use: greater than 99 percent

Implants inserted under your skin are this effective because they take human error off the table. Once it's in, it's in. You personally can't forget to take it and no athletic romp is going to knock it out of place. Some people don't love the idea of a foreign object under their skin—insertion is done only after your skin is numbed, by the way. Once it's in, usually on your upper arm, it releases progestin for up to four years, making this a possible method for people who can't tolerate estrogen. (Actually, the FDA has approved it for three years, research shows it works for four, maybe even five, years, and most providers say four.) Progestin thickens your cervical mucus to help block sperm from getting to an egg. In an implant, it also prevents ovulation. Not loving it or decide you do want to get pregnant after all? Get it removed (this means more numbing agent, a small cut, and it's out). It has a relatively quick return to fertility. It can seem pricey, until you consider the cost over four years. Here's the downside, and keep in mind that this does not happen to all women: the implant may involve irregular bleeding for the first six months to a year. That means spotting or even heavy periods. If this is not OK with you, try another birth control method. Or roll the dice and see how you react; some women say it eventually gives them no period at all. Other less typical complaints include sore breasts and a change in sex drive.

PILL, PATCH, RING

The pill, patch, and the ring are basically the same thing, just administered differently. Functionally they act the same way—the hormones in them are absorbed into your system, are metabolized, then overtake your body's normal cycle and change it. Hormones are administered steadily with the ring and the patch, while with the pill they spike and fall based on when you take your medication. All three methods can be used continuously to suppress periods entirely. And all have pretty similar rebound rates when and if you choose to go off them and try to get pregnant.

– The Patch –

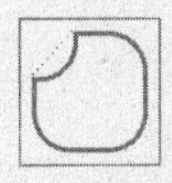

Perfect use: greater than 99 percent

Typical use: 91 percent

The patch is basically a sticker with hormones in it. You adhere it to your skin for three weeks, then take it off for a week if you want to get a period. If not, you use a new patch at week three to suppress your period. Just FYI, if you're looking to avoid your period, you might want a different method. There is a theoretical increased risk of blood clot related to higher exposure to estrogen over time, so some providers are only OK with using the patch for twelve weeks continuously. Overall, the patch is pretty convenient and you don't have to remember to take something daily. You do have to make sure your skin is clean when you stick on a fresh patch—no body lotion, oil, or anything creamy that could keep the patch from adhering. If you have slippery skin, the patch could fall off. If it falls off, just stick it back on (if it's still sticky) or try a new patch. Tape or bandages are not advised. Some women complain the super sticky adhesive gives them a rash or the edges of the patch get a bit grimy as the weeks go by. It can be worn anywhere—butt, back, thigh, arm—but your breasts. It's advisable to choose a comfortable spot where it won't get rubbed—like don't put it where your jeans hug your waist. When you take it off, you're supposed to fold it inward so any remaining hormones on the adhesive won't get out, then throw it away. Side effects can include bleeding between periods, breast soreness, and change in sex drive. Once your body gets used to it, you may see benefits like reduced cramps, lighter periods, and clearer skin (if acne is an issue). If you weigh more than about two hundred pounds, the patch won't work as well for you—your doctor can advise on better, more effective methods. Certain side effects with the patch will be worse if you're a smoker—especially if you're older than thirty-five. Try quitting—and not just because you want to use a patch. You're worth it!

– The Pill –

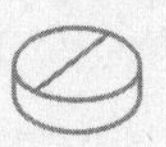

Perfect use: greater than 99 percent

Typical use: 91 percent

The pill is super common—tons of women are on it—but its efficacy drops considerably if you're not someone who can remember to take medication. Dr. Lauren MacAfee says by the third month of use, the typical user misses three or more pills each cycle. Then you wind up doubling or tripling up on missed pills—even if that's not what your doctor would advise—and you get nauseated and vomit because of the extra hormones. Even worse? Misuse and discontinuation of the pill result in a considerable amount of unintended pregnancies. So if you're not someone who is good at taking daily meds, look elsewhere. If you are, give it a try. There are a bunch of kinds of pills on the market, but most of them use a combo of synthetic progesterone (progestin) and estrogen to take over your natural cycle and create its own cycle with lower doses of these hormones. Progestin suppresses ovulation. Estrogen prevents those eggs from developing and getting released. The two of them together change the uterine lining as well as thicken your natural cervical mucus, which helps to block sperm from getting near an egg. There are three weeks of hormones and then a week of placebo pills when you get a period. The pill can be a total goddess send for women with cramps, heavy periods, and acne, especially as it can be taken continuously—if you don't take those placebo pills and just go straight to three more weeks of hormone pills, you won't shed any lining. But the pill can come at a cost: some women report decreased sex drive (see page 77 for why), nausea, and spotting. As with the patch, you shouldn't smoke with the pill. Yet another reason to give up smoking—or to never start. Can't take estrogen? There's a mini pill that's progestin-only and it has no placebo pills. It's tricky, as it requires consistent use—you have to not only take a pill daily but also at the same exact time every day. There are plenty of apps or even the alarm on your phone that can help remind you to take your pill. Sign up for one or set an alarm if you need it—or do both.

– The Ring –

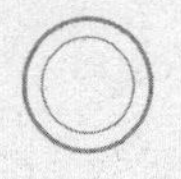

Perfect use: greater than 99 percent

Typical use: 91 percent

The ring is a flexible thing that sort of looks like a rubber bracelet. The hormones are embedded in the ring. They enter your system, preventing your ovaries from releasing eggs and thickening your cervical mucus to block sperm. You wash your hands, then put it in your vagina—really anywhere in your vagina, don't worry you're putting it in the wrong spot. And, no, it can't mistakenly get shoved into your uterus, because your cervix doesn't let stuff pass through like that. (Go back to page 20 and read up on your anatomy!) Worried a partner will feel it? It can be removed for up to three hours—but only once within twenty-four hours. Just. Do. Not. Forget. To. Put. It. Back. In. Or don't take it out for sex, up to you. Other than that, you leave it in place for three weeks and take it out one week a month to get a period. Don't want a period? Wear it continuously, changing to a new ring instead of removing it for a week. It offers the lowest systemic absorption of hormones compared to the patch and the pill, which can help with some of the negative side effects of hormonal birth control. But women wearing rings still report some of the same issues as women on other hormonal methods: bleeding in between periods, sore breasts, nausea, decreased libido. It has the same smoking issue as other hormonal birth control methods—smokers over thirty-five are at increased risk for various side effects. Now for the ring-specific details: it can accidentally be knocked fully out of you when going to the bathroom—especially if you're constipated and pushing super hard. You may not even know it fell out! So be careful. Also, some ring-wearing women report added discharge or even irritation. There are some medical conditions that may mean added risk of blood clots, as with the patch and the pill, but those can be determined by discussing with your doctor and are no reason to rule it out as a method before you have that conversation.

– The Shot –

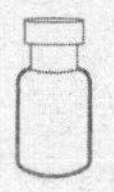

Perfect use: greater than 99 percent

Typical use: 94 percent

Do you hate getting shots? Then this method isn't for you! Don't mind? Well, then consider this: you go to your doctor or a clinic once every three months for a quick shot, and ta-da, you're covered. This is a pretty good deal for women who can't remember to take the pill. But if you're not great about making follow-up appointments, then the shot may not be for you. Some clinics will get in touch with you and help remind you to come in for your shot. If you're late in making an appointment, your doctor may give you a pregnancy test before giving you another shot. The shot contains no estrogen, just synthetic progesterone, which prevents ovulation. Usually it's done in your arm or your butt. If you're thinking about getting pregnant in the near future, you might want to choose another method. Return to fertility with the shot is slow. Women tend to have strong feelings about the shot—some people adore it, some can't handle it. You won't know which camp you fall in or how your body takes to it if you haven't tried it. The positives are clear: it's easy, it's effective, you can forget about it for a few months, and, unlike other more visible methods like the patch or the implant, no one can see or feel you're on it. The negatives are: if you don't like how it makes you feel, you can't go off the shot as quickly as you can other methods; you just have to wait out the three months. Some data shows that the shot is associated with bone mineral density loss, but there's no evidence it increases incidences of fractures. When you go off the shot, research shows bone density returns to what it was. If that concerns you, talk to your doctor. Some women blame the shot for weight gain; irregular bleeding, which can last up to twelve months before evening out and giving most women a lighter period (or no period); loss of libido; depression; and nausea.

OTHER METHODS

Chances are you knew something about everything from condoms to IUDs to the pill. But have you heard about any other methods? You have choices! But let's be clear, if you can't remember to take birth control pills, then something like charting your temperature daily in an effort to be aware of your fertile days probably is not going to be effective at all. Maybe it sounds awesome and you wish you were the type of person who would be that in touch with her own cycle, but we're looking for effectiveness when it comes to birth control, not a wish to be an earthier woman. But if you're meticulous about this sort of thing, then here are some thoughts on alternative birth control methods. Again, these are just the basics. If you're interested in trying one out, do some research before diving in.

– Fertility Awareness Method (FAM) –

Perfect use: 95 to 99 percent

Typical use: 76 to 88 percent

This means learning the ins and outs of your own cycle—the physical signs, symptoms, and other standard data from months of observation—and using them to figure out when you are and are not fertile. You can "read" your cervical mucus and secretions (some kinds indicate ovulation); you can use apps on your phone to help track data; you can use ovulation predictor kits; you can take and make charts of your temperature month by month; you can use a visual aid like CycleBeads. And you can do all these at once. Fertility awareness is not a great idea as your only form of birth control if you have irregular cycles or you're not super in touch with your body or comfortable with your cervix. Yes, you need to know where your cervix is; some women take monthly notes on the position and shape of their cervix. That involves touching it. FAM is not as woo-woo as it sounds. It has real history! And, in modern times, there's an iPhone app to be used with your thermometer—it tracks the data you take. This can truly be effective. In Sweden, one app and thermometer combo has even proved to be more effective than the pill. If you're allergic to spermicide, it's spermicide-free. But you really, really have to be diligent, have to know what you're doing, and, once you do, you have to actually not have sex on your fertile days, which could be a full week—or use great backup. Your partner needs to be down for that, too. If your period is irregular, FAM is not for you. Other pros: it's free, or super low cost for an app and a basal thermometer or ovulation kits, and doesn't require a trip to the doctor. Though you're going to have to pay for a barrier method for the days you think you're fertile. You might want to keep some emergency contraception around in case you have unprotected sex on the wrong day. If you're intrigued, pick up a copy of *Taking Charge of Your Fertility* by Toni Weschler. And don't drop *any* birth control until you know what you're doing!

Breastfeeding

If you've recently had a baby and are breastfeeding exclusively (that means no solids or other liquids are being used, like formula), here's some good news: it can keep you from getting pregnant again! But—and this is a big but—you have to have had no menstrual bleeding since giving birth and you have to be one of those moms who is feeding an under-six-month-old baby around the clock. That means every three to four hours during the day (Planned Parenthood says pumping counts) and every six hours at night. Many women don't even feel too enthused about sex six months after having a baby, but if you fit all the criteria, consider it a gift from nature. And make sure you'd be happy to welcome a sibling, as this method is not hugely effective.

Withdrawal

Failure use is kind of an odd term to use when talking about a guy pulling out before he comes, but to compare it to the other methods here, know that it's 22 percent effective. This is partially because pre-ejaculate can contain sperm and being able to predict exactly when you're going to ejaculate and then getting out of there is actually quite a ninja move. Most people just don't have that sort of mind-body control. If you're going to do it, use a barrier method like spermicide or a cervical cap to up that efficacy rate. And even then, you might want to be prepared for a positive pregnancy test. If you're using condoms exclusively for birth control and want to up their efficacy rate, you could couple pulling out with condoms.

THREE QUESTIONS

1 MY BIRTH CONTROL IS TOTALLY MESSING WITH MY MOOD. WHAT CAN I DO? IT'S LITERALLY DRIVING ME CRAZY!

Call your doctor! Every woman responds to every birth control method in a different way. Your best friend may be rocking the pill or the hormonal IUD no problem, but it's making you totally miserable. Schedule an appointment to go in and then share—no holds barred—what's happening. Is it giving you headaches or cramps or making you never want to have sex? Give your doctor all the details, even if your symptoms are less concrete and more just that you don't feel like you. From there, you can go over all your other choices. It may be that you're not someone who thrives on hormonal birth control. And you'll need to go over all the nonhormonal methods. Their efficacy rates (besides the copper IUD) are not as good as the hormonal methods' rates, so you'll need to talk about ways to increase efficacy. Your doctor may also float the possibility of sticking your current method out. Many women report side effects on new methods that eventually go away or at least calm down as your body gets used to, say, the pill. Hormone levels kind of level off, and then your body feels better. It's totally fine if you're not willing to spend one more month feeling like crap, though. Your body, your decision. Good thing there are plenty of options. Try something else!

2 WHAT'S EMERGENCY BIRTH CONTROL AND HOW DOES IT WORK?

Emergency contraception or EC is what you can take to prevent a pregnancy after unprotected sex but before sperm meets egg. Because there is no embryo, this is not an abortion, nor is it the abortion pill. Accidents happen. Condoms can break or slip off. Someone you think is wearing a condom isn't, or took it off. Drinking or doing drugs might impair good decisions. Maybe you misread your fertility method chart. Perhaps your cervical cap got knocked out of position. And so on. Thankfully there are several methods of contraception available to prevent pregnancy from happening within a certain amount of time *after* unprotected sex. Depending on the type of EC you choose, it can inhibit or delay ovulation, alter sperm motility by thickening cervical mucus, or alter the uterine lining to prevent implantation. Again, these methods are not at all the same thing as the so-called abortion pill; these prevent pregnancy from ever happening in the first place. The abortion pill, on the other hand, is taken any time after a positive pregnancy test for up to ten weeks gestational age—and under the advice of your doctor.

There are several hormonal EC methods available. You can either take an over-the-counter "morning after" pill that's a high dose of synthetic progesterone. It will block or delay ovulation as well as thicken cervical mucus. It's well known as Plan B, widely available, not covered by insurance, and is usually around fifty dollars. Some states have rules about women under eighteen purchasing it. You need to take this within seventy-two hours of having sex and carefully follow the directions given to you by the pharmacist. Or you can call your doctor—time is of the essence, don't delay picking up your phone! There is one kind of morning-after pill that requires a prescription. It's called Ella and is highly effective, particularly for overweight women, and can be used within five days after sex. Or your gyno can walk you through taking higher than normal doses of certain birth control pills. Taking extra amounts of an estrogen and progesterone combo pill as outlined by your doctor will also delay ovulation. The extra estrogen does tend to make some women nauseous. Another option your doctor may suggest is having a copper IUD inserted within five days after unprotected sex. It will do what it always does—impair any sperm that do make it to your uterus as well as create an inhospitable environment for implantation. This is also the only option that will provide ongoing pregnancy prevention going forward—win-win.

3 I'M TRYING TO DECIDE WHAT KIND OF BIRTH CONTROL TO USE. WHEN I READ ABOUT ALL THE SIDE EFFECTS, IT SOUNDS LIKE A LOT OF THEM MAKE YOU SPOT. WHAT, EXACTLY, IS SPOTTING? I MEAN, I KNOW IT'S BLOOD COMING OUT THAT ISN'T A FULL PERIOD, BUT WHY DOES IT HAPPEN?

You got it—spotting is breakthrough bleeding. You are most likely to spot when you're first on a specific birth control as your body gets used to the new-to-you hormones. And you're more likely to spot if you have chosen birth control with little or no estrogen—the hormonal IUD, the shot, the implant, the mini pill, or a pill with low estrogen. That's because estrogen, among other things, stabilizes the lining of your uterus. When you have less of it, that uterine lining can shed a little, which you see as spots of blood in your underwear. If spotting is bothering you, you can either give it a few months until your body gets used to the birth control, or you can switch to another method—something with more estrogen, or a non-hormonal birth control. Call your gynecologist, who may have other ideas for you. If you're spotting and *not* on a low- or no-estrogen birth control method, a call to your doc is also in order. Spotting can signal a few things, including an infection or maybe an STI, or even pregnancy.

CHAPTER 5

SAFER SEX IS GREAT SEX:

HOW AND WHY TO PROTECT YOURSELF

Sex is great, but not if you're being unsafe about it. If you're getting it on, you need to protect yourself and your partner from a whole bunch of infections and diseases. And yet only 21 percent of sexually active women ages twenty to forty-four use condoms regularly (!!!). This literally makes no sense. Women are taking care of their health. They're working out. They're trying to sleep more and eat better. Some of them drink green juice and go to yoga. They smoke less and less. They're more in touch with their mental health. So why would they be having unprotected sex? Let's say this once, and then over and over again: having safer sex is taking care of your health in the best possible way. It's getting on top.

Back when HIV and AIDS were still relatively newish, a generation of people became sexually active knowing that unsafe sex could mean death. We're far enough removed from that time that many young people no longer see HIV and AIDS as an immediate threat to their health. Maybe they're feeling invincible. But here's the thing: we are not invincible. There is a host of diseases—some far more serious than others—that anyone, including you, can contract through vaginal, oral, or anal sex. And you do not want them! The only way to avoid STIs entirely is not to have sex. But that's not how most women want to live their lives. So you need to have safer sex. For women or men who have sex with men, this means condoms are nonnegotiable. They're a fact of life. Also, you need to get tested for STIs even if you use condoms—on the reg. Many of us are walking around carrying STIs but have no symptoms, so we don't even know we have—and are spreading—diseases. And while you're at it, insist on partners who also like safe sex and sharing test results. Knowledge is power.

Sexually transmitted infections are frighteningly common, like common cold common. The CDC says one in four sexually active adolescent females have an STI. Young people—adolescents and young adults—are more likely to be exposed (though older people, including divorcées and widows not familiar with safer sex practices, are busily catching up!). The CDC says that while people ages fifteen to twenty-four make up around one-quarter of all sexually active people, they also account for half of the twenty million new STIs that happen in the United States yearly. And though the prevalence of casual sex in this dating-app moment might make it feel otherwise, some STIs are on the rise. The CDC says between 2010 and 2014, gonorrhea cases went up by more than 90 percent. Syphilis and chlamydia are also up—the former by about 65 percent in that same time frame while the latter increased by around 52 percent in adults sixty-five and older. Young women may be more susceptible to infection because of something called cervical ectopy. This is when cells usually located within the cervix are on the outside, a normal finding in adolescent and young women. This, plus the various barriers young women face when accessing reproductive health care, is a bad combo.

It's not about limiting your sexual partners. You can clearly contract an STI with just one partner—even in a monogamous relationship if a partner isn't exhibiting signs of a disease they are carrying. It only takes one encounter to contract an infection. Truth. One bad decision and you could have a disease for life. We need to understand the gravity of this and to know we all have the choice to protect ourselves. Bacteria and viruses do not know or care about how many partners you have had—they just want a warm body to inhabit. Most sexually transmitted infections are treatable with no lasting repercussions, while other diseases can lead to infertility and even shorten your life. If you haven't been great about practicing safer sex until reading this very sentence, no judgment. Just commit now to practicing safer sex and to going to the doctor frequently for exams and STI screenings.

When you go for testing, be honest with your doctor about what you have been up to, including if you've had a lot of partners. Are you swinging? Share the news. Many doctors only screen for HIV, so you should ask what they test for and discuss if you should be tested for more than just HIV. You want to know what's happening with your health, like if you're carrying an undetected disease with no outward symptoms.

STIs are yet another reason it's important to have a good working relationship with your own vagina. If you know what it's like when it's healthy—what it looks like, what it smells like—you'll be more likely to notice when something's off. You'll recognize an unusual discharge or scent or itch or sore. Ob-gyn Dr. Angela says a lot of people show up in her office thinking something is an ingrown hair that is certainly not an ingrown hair! Yes, vulvas are bumpy-looking, but there's a big difference between the skin on the labia and a regular run-of-the-mill pimple and a herpes sore. If you feel or see anything unusual, take your vagina in to be looked at.

Keep in mind that STIs can be passed by fluid (precum, semen, vaginal fluid, blood) but also by skin-to-skin contact. Barriers like condoms, used correctly, block the fluid, but they cannot entirely prevent skin contact as they don't cover all of the genital area. This does not mean you should not have sex. By all means, have sex! Just be safe.

CONDOMS: THE ULTIMATE SEXUAL PARTNER

You can avoid STIs in several ways. First, no sex at all. Second, be in a long-term, mutually monogamous relationship with an uninfected partner who has been thoroughly tested (lots of infected people are unaware of their infections because they don't know they have one and are not exhibiting symptoms). Third, consistent and correct use of latex condoms (see page 112 on how to use condoms effectively). The CDC says this means male condoms, and Planned Parenthood says the female condom also helps. Either way, avoid condoms made of lamb-skin. Yes, they can protect against pregnancy, but they contain tiny pores and therefore do not protect against STIs. Think about it this way: every safer sexual encounter is a three-way—you, your partner, and a condom. Anatomically, condoms cannot cover all the skin that could potentially transmit an STI like herpes or HPV, like the base of the penis and the balls, but they're as good as we've got. Condoms are particularly good for protection against STIs transmitted by fluids, like gonorrhea, chlamydia, trichomoniasis, and HIV infection. We know this because their use has been amply studied. Research has proven latex condoms provide an effective barrier against even the smallest disease pathogens. And condoms have even been extensively tested for efficacy in relationships where one part-

SAFER SEX, DEFINED

This is what it means to have safer sex (there's no such thing as 100 percent safe sex).

USE BARRIERS. Condoms, dental dams, even latex gloves. Every single time you have oral, vaginal, or anal sex. Don't gloss over the word *oral*! Wrap it up for blow jobs, and use dental dams when you go down or someone goes down on you. And use those gloves for whatever you're up to manually.

DON'T SHARE. Sharing is caring, just not when it comes to sex toys. Only share if you've properly cleaned your toys. And remember: toys can wear condoms, too. It's a good idea. When you're done, put a new condom on the toy before sharing.

KEEP IT CLEAN. This includes your hands.

VISIT YOUR DOCTOR. This should at least be a yearly event, but if you're someone who has a lot of sexual partners, go more often. You cannot eyeball someone's genitals, see no warts or sores, and think you are good to go unprotected and have not been exposed. That's not how STIs work or how they always present. Only professionals plus tests can "read" bodies for disease.

CHOOSE PARTNERS WHO VISIT THEIR DOCTORS. Whether you're randomly hooking up or taking your time to get to know one specific person, ask about their latest STI testing and overall sexual health history and status. Test results need to be recent and comprehensive; certain infections can lie dormant and many people don't even know they're infected, because they're asymptomatic and unrecognized—all the more reason to use condoms. And be transparent in sharing your test results, too. Someone who does not want to have this conversation is probably not someone you want intimately involved with your body.

MAKE SMART CHOICES. You know what's not a great idea by now: unprotected sex, including oral, and especially anal. Just don't do it. And don't do nonsexual things that could expose you to STIs, either, like sharing needles for IV drugs or going to unclean tattoo parlors. Safeguard your health and your amazing body.

MASTURBATION IS AWESOME. Just met someone who is totally hot? Penetrative sex doesn't need to be a given; neither does oral. Pretend you're in high school but with a lot more knowledge about how your body gets off, then go at it, mutually. Win-win.

ner is HIV-infected and the other is not. So we know consistent use is both critical and works.

CONDOM 101

A condom is basically a tight-fitting latex glove for a penis. While a small number of condoms are made from other materials like animal intestines or polyurethane, the vast majority of condoms are made from latex. Latex may sound like it's synthetic, and some is, but 100 percent of latex used in condoms is actually natural—made from the sap of rubber trees. The trees get tapped, a milky substance comes out, and this gets manufactured into latex. Latex is put over molds of various shapes and sizes and that's how condoms are made.

Condoms are controlled by the FDA as a class II medical device. This classification is meant to ensure that all condoms sold in the United States adhere to particular performance standards—no matter what the brand. And the FDA requires certain tests that seek out holes or areas of thinning to ensure quality and performance. All condoms, thick or thin, must meet the same FDA reliability and safety standards. As for lubricated condoms, the FDA currently allows only one lubricant to be used inside the foil wrapper and that's silicone—a man-made polymer. So if you're the kind of person who prefers organic to petroleum lube, you're not going to find it inside condom packaging—not yet, anyway. But you can, of course, seek out organic for any extra lubricant you might want.

The differences between condom brands usually come down to shapes, texture, and ingredients. Just to be clear here, *any* condom is always better than no condom. Period. So what kind of condom should you carry? If you don't have a regular partner, it's good to be prepared for just about anything—so your best bet is an option that's meant to fit the majority of men. After you've selected the size, you want to consider how thin or thick it is. A thin condom could increase sensitivity and sensation, while a thicker condom could help prolong the proceedings and make a man last longer—it all depends on the guy, so why not ask for their input. And finally, decide if you want texture that could increase sensations for you and your partner.

Shapes

Penises come in all different sizes, but people purchasing condoms tend to upsize, buying ones that are too big for them or their partners. It turns out only 10 to 15 percent of the population actually requires a larger fit. As in, chances are you don't need them. If you're buying condoms to use on sex toys, you also won't need them. You might need a dictionary to wade through some of the fantastic terms various companies have come up with for the generic words *small*, *medium*, and *large*. But basically you get the gist. The sizes only apply to girth, not length, by the way. If your partner isn't comfortable in his current condom, keep testing different fits, shapes, and sizes until you find perfection.

Texture

To rib or not to rib. Only you and your partner know the answer. Try a few different textures out and, if you and your partner like them, and actually feel a difference or added sexual sensation, then by all means keep using them! Studs, dots, or otherwise, they make no difference in terms of efficacy. Some of those bumps and tickles are supposed to stimulate women, others are for men, some work for both. If textured condoms do nothing extra special for you, the experimenting trial phase will at the very least be a fun game for all involved.

Ingredients

The FDA doesn't require condom manufacturers to list or disclose their ingredients to consumers. In the absence of ingredient lists, here's what we do know about what's in condoms: Some natural latex condoms can contain by-products called nitrosamines—these are carcinogenic chemicals that form when liquid latex is heated up to the point at which it becomes solid and an accelerator is added to the mix to speed up the process. Bodily fluids can cause nitrosamines to be released from the latex while you're having sex. If you don't want carcinogenic chemicals in or around your vagina, choose a brand that has no detectable levels of nitrosamines in the finished product. This should be called out on the product packaging. Always read labels. Beyond nitrosamines, some condoms can have other chemicals of concern in them including fragrance, flavor chemicals, and spermicide. If you don't want things like this in your vagina that could irritate it and mess with its pH, buy and carry your own condoms that don't contain them. Look for claims of scents and flavors on the packaging so you can avoid them. Remember, vaginal irritation can make you more at risk for an STI, which totally defeats the purpose.

The Extras

Beyond ingredients, size, and texture, when shopping for condoms, you can also keep an eye out for all kinds of extras that might appeal to you, too. Some are manufactured in more eco-friendly ways than others. Are you pro–fair trade and anti–child labor? Look for a condom that's fair-trade certified. Are you vegan? Then you'll want a condom that's third-party certified vegan. Most condoms have a dairy by-product called casein in them, but a vegan condom would not. Are you allergic to latex? You'll need to seek out nonlatex condoms.

A few other friendly reminders as you shop: lube—used with condoms—is great for increasing female pleasure and helping men last longer. Add it to your regimen. But do not use body oil or gels as lubricants; they can potentially destroy the latex. Always go for water- or silicone-based lubricant. And, once you've made your pick, never ever reuse a condom. And throw them in the garbage after every use; they should not be flushed.

ORAL SEX

In terms of contracting diseases, oral—blow jobs, cunnilingus, and analingus—is statistically somewhat safer than anal or vaginal sex. But it's still possible to get an infection from unprotected oral, even if you only do it briefly as part of foreplay before penetration. Unprotected oral is especially risky if you have a compromised immune system and/or bleeding gums or sores in your mouth. You may even have a cut in your mouth you're not aware of. What does this mean in practice? If you go down on someone who is HIV positive, you can get HIV—though oral transmission of HIV is pretty rare. You can contract gonorrhea in your throat. You can wind up at higher risk for HPV-related oral cancer. And if you yourself have a herpes sore in your mouth and go down on someone with no barrier, you can give that person genital herpes.

Basically pretty much any STI can be transmitted orally and yet, anecdotally, people are totally not using condoms or dental dams on the reg for oral. Part of the issue is that

SO YOU WANT TO STOP USING CONDOMS?

Here's the sitch: You're in a long-term monogamous relationship and you and your partner mutually agree you'd like to get rid of the condoms. That word *mutually* is key here; if you want to keep using condoms but your partner does not or vice versa, you have to have some real conversations on how best to arrive at a plan you both agree on. Give yourself some time as you make this decision. Getting rid of barrier protection—even if neither of you has tested positive for an STI and even if you are both truly only having sex with each other—always involves some risk. STIs could emerge, previously undetected in your bloodstream. It happens. Or you may have oral herpes and spread it via unprotected oral sex. That's why pulling condoms from your sex life is a big-deal decision. It has to be made together and must be rooted in trust and honesty.

Before you finalize your plan, there are a few things you'll want to do. First up, go get tested for STIs. Do a *full* workup, even the stuff doctors might not normally test for, and have your partner do the same. Keep in mind that recent infections won't automatically show up on these tests. So if one or both of you has been with other people in the not-so-distant past, keep in mind that you might want to repeat the testing at an interval determined by you and your doctor. Then share results. Don't forget to ask and share if you've been vaccinated for any STIs like HPV and hepatitis. Next, you'll want to make sure that you both agree on what monogamy means. Some couples are fine with a little side play, but you need to spell out what that translates to in terms of mutual protection against STIs. Complete transparency is key in terms of keeping healthy. When you've agreed on that, plus the results are in from your tests and you're both healthy, then do as you wish. Just don't forget birth control if you're not prepared to have a baby.

the education around safe sex is mostly focused on far riskier anal and vaginal sex, so safer oral isn't as talked about. But it's good common sense. What's the hang-up? Why is it any better or worse to lick or suck through latex than have it on you or in you, especially considering what it can protect you against? It's a smart idea, so give it a try. And if you meet any resistance with your partner, well, then, they just don't get serviced. Their loss. Flavored condoms may or may not make it tastier for you to suck on latex—pretend it's a lollipop? And if you don't have a dental dam but you do have a condom, it's easy to turn into a dental dam—just cut off the tip and that bottom ring, then cut straight up the middle to make a rectangle. Cover that over the vulva or asshole as a barrier. Then do your thing.

A TO Z: INFECTIONS AND DISEASES

Here's a list of most of the STIs currently out there. Even if you're not feeling bad, get tested at least yearly; you may have something with no symptoms, and when some STIs go untreated for long periods of time they can mess with your reproductive system and ultimately lead to infertility. The following is *general* information. If you have an STI, you'll want to do your own research that goes beyond these basics.

There are many solid resources, from Planned Parenthood to the CDC (where a lot of the information that follows comes from) to the Guttmacher Institute, among others. Check them out. To minimize your chances of ever getting any of the infections listed below, use condoms. If you're treating a current infection, ask your doctor if you should be refraining from sexual activity until you're better. And just because an STI is treatable right now does not mean it will remain that way. There are diseases currently on the rise that are becoming increasingly resistant to most classes of antibiotics used to fight them. Serious stuff.

One caveat: this list isn't exhaustive. It's missing a few diseases, like mono (which you can get from kissing and without having sex but some people still consider it an STI), Zika (which is mainly spread through a mosquito bite, though can be shared through unprotected sex, and is most risky for women who are already pregnant or in the process of getting pregnant), and canchroid (a bacterial infection that causes open sores around your genitals and is rarely seen in the United States but is something to know about if you travel a lot and are planning on having fun at your destination). Always be up on the latest STIs so you can take steps to protect yourself. And don't let any of this freak you out or shut you down. Sex is such a key part of a full life—just stay safe out there.

CHLAMYDIA

WHAT IS IT? The most common bacterial STI reported to the CDC, chlamydia is spread through vaginal, anal, or oral sex, plus shared sex toys and even childbirth (a mother can pass it to her child). A man does not have to ejaculate to spread it. Young people are at higher risk than others for contracting chlamydia based on behaviors like not using condoms and increased number of partners. It can infect men and women. Many people who have contracted it don't even know they have it, as it doesn't always have symptoms. If you do have symptoms, typically they are abnormal vaginal discharge and a burning sensation when peeing, plus painful sex, swelling, cervical pain, and sometimes nausea or fever. In women, it infects the cervix and can spread up through the reproductive system and ultimately cause infertility. It's associated with pelvic inflammatory disease as well as ectopic pregnancy (that's when a fertilized egg implants outside the uterus and isn't viable). If you contract it in your ass, you'd have pain there, discharge, and possibly bleeding. For men, it infects the urethra, and similarly can spread into the reproductive system and cause infertility, though that's rare.

TEST: Lab tests are done from urine or swab samples of the genital area.

TREATMENT: Antibiotics. Once you're cured, you're not immune to catching chlamydia again in the future, even from your current partner. It's actually very easy for couples to reinfect each other. So you have to refrain from sex until you're both clear, and you may even want to retest in a few months just to make sure. Also, you'll need to get in touch with anyone you were sexually active with within a two-month stretch to let them know to get treated pronto. That might be awkward, but, considering the long-term possible health effects of chlamydia, honesty is the best policy.

GONORRHEA

WHAT IS IT? The CDC says there are more than eight hundred thousand new cases of gonorrhea, often called the clap, reported yearly, making it the second-most reported bacterial STI in the United States. It's likely underreported, as many people don't have symptoms, so they don't bother to get tested. You get it by having sex (vaginal, anal, oral) with someone who is infected. Pregnant mothers can also pass it to their babies during childbirth. It's super common with young people, ages fifteen to twenty-four. It causes infections in genitals plus your ass and throat. Most women don't have symptoms, or have mild ones like unexplained vaginal or anal discharge or general itchiness, soreness, bleeding between periods, or pain, including painful

TESTING FOR ALL

If you're having sex regularly, you should be tested for STIs regularly. This is best for your health, obviously, but also this way you'll know if you're carrying anything that you're spreading around unknowingly. There are so many different ways to get tested these days. The choices are bountiful—both free and paid. You can go to your doctor's office, visit a local health clinic, or find a same-day testing center. There are even apps that let you make profiles and order certain kinds of tests online, and have them shipped discreetly to your door. App results are easy to share with partners or even as part of your public profile on a dating site. Some sites block users from sharing test results if they've tested positive for a disease until they've been treated, been tested again, and are clear of disease. Other apps allow HIV-positive people to share the level of HIV in their blood.

Any test is better than no test, just to be clear. If you can, the best place to get tested is at a trusted health center—this could be your local clinic or your own personal doctor. A urine test is easy enough to take at home, but some diseases are better detected via a blood sample or a visual inspection. Seeing someone in person also tends to mean access to the most up-to-date tests preferred by the medical community administered by people who deal with these tests all day long. And you get results IRL with someone there to provide reassurance, support, and a plan of action if you do test positive. If going to a clinic isn't an option for you, and you use an at-home test that results in a positive test, you'll get digital information on what you need to do to treat your disease—including scheduling an in-person appointment if necessary.

If you test negative, but you know you have had a risky encounter within a short time frame, test again to make sure you're truly negative. Some infections take longer than others to incubate. Your age and your sexual activity will dictate which tests your health care provider gives you, based on some very general recommendations by the CDC. Speak up if you want something specific tested for, as your own behavior may not fit with such generalizations.

poops. These are all easily confused with other vaginal and anal infections. This is unfortunate, as gonorrhea puts women at risk for infertility, pelvic inflammatory disease, and ectopic pregnancy, and can increase the risk of getting or transmitting HIV. For men, the symptoms can include having to pee a lot, and urgently; discharge from the penis; pain with or without swelling in the testicles; a red or swollen penis opening; and a sore throat.

TEST: Usually just a urine sample. You can also test with a swab of your ass, throat, or genitals. Occasionally you need more swabbing—of your cervix or, for men, of their urethra (via the pee hole).

TREATMENT: Antibiotics, again, to the rescue. Want to hear something terrifying? Gonorrhea has been progressively developing resistance to the drugs used to treat it. That means the germs don't respond and continue to multiply. The CDC calls this an "urgent public health issue" and the medical community is working on finding future medications to combat the disease. For now, there are still drugs that work, so if you have gonorrhea and take them, you will likely be completely cured. But, as with chlamydia, repeat infections are common in couples continuing to have unprotected sex. So lay off it while you're going through treatment and be honest with your partners about your status.

TREATMENT FOR TWO

Back in 2006, the CDC said doctors who treat patients for STIs like chlamydia and gonorrhea should also provide treatment for the patient's partner, even if that person isn't their patient and even if they never came into the office for testing. This is called "expedited partner therapy," and it makes so much sense. It can drastically reduce reinfection rates, which are pretty high. Currently, some states have laws and regulations supporting partner therapy; others don't. If you or your partner has been diagnosed with an STI, check out what the rules are in your state. You may just save yourself a trip to the doc.

HEPATITIS

WHAT IS IT? There are actually several kinds of hepatitis. All are infectious viruses that can harm the liver (*hepatitis* means inflammation of the liver)—sometimes very seriously. Hepatitis A, B, and C are most common, but B is the one that's most commonly considered an STI. Technically all can be shared through sex partners. B can be transmitted through body fluids (blood, semen, vaginal discharge, etc.), either through sexual contact or through sharing of needles. It can also be transmitted from moms to babies at birth. C is considered a blood-borne virus and is not effectively transmitted via sex, though the CDC says there is data indicating it can be sexually transmitted, especially with people who also have HIV. A is typically spread through a fecal-oral route, like via contaminated food or water, but it could occur through oral-anal contact. Symptoms depend on which kind of hep you have, and many people have no symptoms. If you do feel something, it's likely to feel similar to the flu—fever, aches, exhaustion, maybe nausea, and vomiting.

TEST: Blood test at your doctor's office or a lab.

TREATMENT: Prevention is better than treatment. There are vaccines for A and B (most kids are now vaccinated against both as part of routine shots), so look into those and make sure you're up to date. Antibodies produced in response to hepatitis A last for life and protect against reinfection. Long-term hep B is usually related to what age you are at infection. Babies are more likely to be chronically infected than adults. C is more likely than A or B to become a long-term, chronic infection.

HERPES

WHAT IS IT? Our friend Dr. Angela says herpes is like roaches; the virus has been around for eternity and no one can eradicate it. There are two kinds of herpes—simplex type 1 and simplex type 2. Type 1 is incredibly common. You know you have it if you get cold sores on your mouth. Type 2 is the one that's usually below the belt. But guess what? Type 1 is heading south at a speedy rate thanks to young people who have oral sex (which is great) but mainly go at it unprotected (not so great). We're all for an uptick in oral sex—especially reciprocal oral—but this is an unfortunate side effect, because herpes lasts forever. It's also super common. The CDC says one in six people aged fourteen to forty-nine in the United States has genital herpes. Part of why it's so virulent is that many people who carry it don't have visible symptoms either on their junk or on their mouth. And it doesn't always flare up in a body immediately after exposure. Yes, it's most contagious when there is a visibly active or angry-looking sore, but it can spread with no visible sores, too. You could come into contact with it through kissing, oral sex, and/or genital contact and not see outbreaks until later in life. And it's not always spread sexually. Pregnant moms can pass it to their babies, which can be potentially dangerous.

When it comes to genital exposure, herpes can be shared even without fluid sharing. Say you're messing around and genital skin is touching and rubbing other genital skin before you put on a condom. That could do it. Herpes just needs contact between an infected area of one body and an uninfected area on another body. Usually it's an area with skin like the mouth or the vagina, but also incudes butts, vulvas, and penises.

The most obvious symptoms are sores—on your mouth (cold sores or fever blisters) or on your genitals, plus possibly up in your vagina or even on your cervix. If your symptoms are mild, you may think a sore is just an ingrown hair or a random rash or bump. They are not. These may or may not give you a tingling sensation prior to outbreak. They're usually pretty painful, especially during the first outbreak. And they are reoccurring, especially in the first year after exposure. You might also experience fever, swollen glands, pain when peeing, unusual discharge, or bleeding between periods.

TEST: Doctors will culture a lesion if one is present and can test your blood to determine if you have been exposed to herpes in the past.

TREATMENT: Once you have herpes, you have it for life. There's a medication for reducing the number of outbreaks you experience as well as the risk of transmission to a partner. Depending on how frequent your outbreaks are, you may take this very rarely. Or, if you have a lot of outbreaks, or if your immune system is compromised, you may want to take it daily as a preventative measure. Your doctor will help you decide which route to go. If you have herpes or are sleeping with someone who does, be honest with your partners, and then use barriers and safer sex techniques. This lowers but doesn't completely get rid of the risk. Never touch an open sore with your hand; it can easily be transferred to another part of your body, including your eyes. If you do, wash your hands well. If you have open sores and are sexually active, this puts you at a higher risk for getting or giving HIV (if you have it).

HPV

WHAT IS IT? Human papillomavirus wins the dubious award of being the most common STI in the United States. Nearly all sexually active people get it at some point in their lives. It's that prevalent. The CDC says about seventy-nine million Americans are currently infected with HPV and about fourteen million people become newly infected each year. There are multiple strains of HPV and some of them don't do anything bad to you. HPV can resolve itself. But if you have a "bad" strain, and it doesn't go away on its own, it can lead to genital warts and even cancer in both men and women (cervical, vaginal, anal, penile, and oral). It's unclear why and how certain strains resolve themselves. This is why the CDC currently suggests routine HPV vaccination, for both girls and boys, starting as young as age eleven. At the moment, the vaccine only covers some strains, and it takes three vaccines over a set period of time to be protected. The idea in starting that young is to be fully protected before sexual contact and potential exposure begins. If you start vaccination older than that, it will not protect you from prior exposure. If you're unvaccinated and interested in getting vaccinated, talk to your doctor. The CDC's recommendations based on age and sexual activity have changed as the vaccine gets further developed, so check their website, too.

HPV is spread through sexual contact—vaginal, anal, oral, as well as manual. And it can be spread through exposed skin, not just penetration or sharing of fluids. This means condoms are important but cannot entirely protect you as they don't cover all of the genitals. Some active strains will produce warts on genitals, but usually there are no visible symptoms. Even without warts, HPV can still be present and contagious.

TEST: The test most frequently used for HPV is the Pap smear. This is a lifesaving diagnostic tool that screens for cervical cancer, which is associated with HPV. There's a separate HPV test that can show what specific HPV strains you might have and is sometimes used in conjunction with a Pap smear. Chances are you've already had at least one Pap smear—great. It involves scraping some cells off your cervix then looking at them for precancerous conditions caused by some strains of HPV. Get yours on the reg. There is no similar test for men—HPV can only be detected if there are visible warts. Those can be sampled, but currently there is no HPV test routinely recommended for men. However, some experts suggest anal Pap tests for gay, bisexual, and HIV-positive men since anal cancer is more common for them.

TREATMENT: Some strains may resolve themselves, some will not. If you're unvaccinated, talk to your doctor about whether the vaccine still makes sense for you. If you have warts, you can have them removed—but you will still have HPV. If you don't remove them, they either stay the same, go away, or grow in number. The best treatment is prevention and safer sex. Make sure to get your Pap smears consistently so you can treat whatever is found nice and early before it becomes cancer. It can take a number of years after HPV exposure to develop cancer. If you know you have HPV, share this information with your partner. If you have it, they will likely have it, too. It's that contagious.

HIV/AIDS

WHAT IS IT? Human immunodeficiency virus (HIV) is a potentially deadly STI that attacks the immune system and weakens the body's ability to fight disease, including run-of-the-mill illnesses like a cold. AIDS stands for acquired immunodeficiency syndrome—it's a condition that can develop if you are HIV positive. HIV is spread through body fluids (blood, semen, even breast milk) and is the most dangerous STI, since currently there is no vaccine and no effective cure for it. According to the CDC's most recent statistics from 2014, there were an estimated 37,600 new HIV infections (down from 45,700 in 2008), and an estimated 1.1 million people in the United States are living with HIV. Of those people, one in seven don't even know they're infected. Anyone of any age, race, sex, or sexual orientation can be infected—everyone from young women of color to gay men and everywhere in between. The main risk factor? Unprotected sex—anal or vaginal. Risk increases with multiple sexual partners. Risk increases if you have another STI. Sores can act as a path for HIV to enter your body. Risk increases if you use IV drugs. Risk also increases if you're an uncircumcised male.

After HIV exposure, some people report flulike or mono-like symptoms, but not everyone experiences these. Many of the symptoms related to HIV can easily be mistaken for other diseases: mouth sores, yeast infections, exhaustion, stiffness of joints.

Condoms, properly used, are the most important tool in preventing HIV. Using water- or silicone-based lubricants can help keep the condoms from slipping or breaking. Never use oil-based lubes, as they can weaken the latex. Avoid spermicides in the lubricant; they can irritate the lining of both your vagina and ass. Irritated skin increases the risk of exposure. Additionally, you can modify your sexual behavior to avoid the most risky acts. As in: anal sex, especially receptive anal sex, is high risk because the lining of your ass is thin and prone to tearing, making space for HIV to enter your bloodstream. Oral sex is less risky. Also key to lowering your risk of exposure: avoiding contact with blood and urine, especially with your mouth, ass, eyes, and any cuts or sores you might have. Avoiding sexual activity with partners who use IV drugs is a good idea. If you're sexually active, routine testing for HIV is a must.

TEST: Your doctor will check either blood or oral fluid. There are various kinds of tests, including anonymous (only you will know the results) and confidential (your results will become part of your medical record). Some tests are rapid and you can get results as you wait. Your doctor will explain to you what you need to know about the window of time between exposure and when HIV is detectable in your system. You'll want to screen at least yearly if not more often, depending on your sex life. A negative test does not mean you can discontinue actions to prevent HIV if you're sexually active. Honesty is critical when it comes to HIV status. If you're positive, you must let partners—past, present, and future—know.

TREATMENT: There is no cure, but HIV can be controlled with good medical care that includes antiviral drugs plus self-care to keep your immune system as strong as possible. Avoiding illness can slow the trajectory of the disease from HIV to AIDS. There is near-constant research being done on HIV. If you have it, you will want to work with an HIV specialist to have access to the best and newest medications. There is also prescription medication—Truvada for PrEP—that can reduce the risk of getting an HIV infection when combined with safer sex practices. If you're at high risk for HIV through partners or IV drug use, speak to your doctor about it. Keep in mind medication is not magic and should never be considered a replacement for proper condom use and routine testing.

ITCHY STUFF

WHAT IS IT? Oh, pubic lice and scabies, would that all STIs be this tiny, annoying, and no big deal to cure! Lice are parasitic mites, aka crabs, that get in your pubes and feed on your blood. When you have sex, they can take a ride over to your partner's pubes, even if you're using a condom. You could also actually get them from a roommate or even at the gym, as they can live on things like damp towels (don't share towels!). If you've got them, speak up so others don't borrow your towel. Scabies are another kind of tiny parasites that infect the top layer of your skin and cause super itchy rashes. It's pretty gross to consider mites under your skin laying eggs. They spread easily if skin touches skin, especially during sex or even just sleeping in the same bed with someone, and are considered a skin condition. Thankfully it's rare to get them from casual touching.

TEST: You kind of know it if you have pubic lice, but if you want to know what's making you itchy, your doc can take a skin sample and check it out under a microscope. Usually your doc will be able to make a visual call regarding if you have scabies.

TREATMENT: For crabs, there are over-the-counter shampoos and lotions—read ingredients to try to use the least harsh ones available. Then do a serious wash of clothes, sheets, towels, etc. in super-crazy-hot water. Try not to scratch if you can; you're likely to take that same hand and accidentally transfer the mites to your head or even your eyelashes. Ack! Scabies can make you uncomfy, but medicated creams and sometimes pills can help—so you'll need to take your itchy self to the doctor for a prescription. They take a little while to clear the itching and totally get rid of the parasites. You'll also need to do a total detox of clothes, towels, and bedding for scabies. Vacuuming may also be in order. Make sure your partner is being treated at the same time so you don't reinfect each other.

SYPHILIS

WHAT IS IT? This old-school bacterial infection was at one point on the decline but now is rising again. It's usually spread through all kinds of sexual contact, typically via a sore on or around the penis, vagina, ass (it could be inside the vagina and the ass, too), or even on the lips and in the mouth. If you don't treat it, you could wind up with neurosyphilis, which can really mess with your nervous system. Untreated syphilis can also lead to organ damage and loss of eyesight. In severe cases, it can kill you. Babies born to mothers with syphilis can have both mental and physical problems, which is why ob-gyns typically test pregnant moms for it. It's not the easiest disease to diagnose. Many of its symptoms are similar to other diseases. Or you may have no symptoms at all. It's a disease that doctors consider in four stages and it presents differently in each one. For the primary stage, look for ulcers one to six weeks after exposure. These are basically a skin rash of one or more coin-size sores and can transmit the disease. They aren't usually painful, and they are firm. Because they don't hurt, many people never see them or overlook them as nothing to register. You might also have flulike symptoms. Condoms work well for blocking access to sores in the areas they can cover, but sometimes sores appear outside of their area of coverage. If you're sexually active, you should test for syphilis yearly, especially since you might not know you're carrying it. Statistically speaking, getting tested is especially important for men who have sex with men.

TEST: A doctor can do a microscopic examination of fluid from any sores present or a blood test.

TREATMENT: Antibiotics (typically penicillin) for all! That's you and any of your partners, to prevent reinfection. If you treat in the disease's early stages, this will do the trick and cure you. Don't forgo treatment just because a sore goes away—that can happen, but it does not mean you don't have the disease. And keep getting tested; just because you had it once does not mean you can't get it again.

TRICHOMONIASIS

WHAT IS IT? Trichomoniasis, or trich, is a fairly common parasite that spreads easily during sex, including manual stimulation, through precum, semen, and vaginal fluids. Lots of people have it, especially under the age of thirty-five, but they won't know because they have no symptoms. Planned Parenthood says about seven out of ten people with trich have no signs of the infection. When it does present symptoms, they are ones that can seem like other diseases including vaginitis (irritated vulva or vagina), an infection of your urethra (you know, the tube connecting your bladder to your pee hole), frequent or painful peeing, and stinky discharge. Men don't usually present symptoms but can still have it. Trich can also be spread through sex toys, damp towels, and bathing suits, so these are best not shared. Thankfully it cannot be transmitted casually—like through hugging or even from toilet seats. Condoms are solid for preventing trich.

TEST: Your doctor will look at your discharge under a microscope and do a genital exam and will be able to say, "Hey this is trich," and not a UTI or chlamydia or anything else you might think it feels like.

TREATMENT: Antibiotics to the rescue for you and your sex partner (yes, both of you need to be treated to avoid reinfection). Your doc may tell you that you should avoid sex for the duration of the treatment.

PELVIC INFLAMMATORY DISEASE

WHAT IS IT? Pelvic inflammatory disease, or PID, is a bacterial infection of the uterus, uterine lining, tubes, and ovaries. It's not technically an STI; it can't be contagious, but you get it from STIs (usually). If you're interested in having children at some point in life, PID is a real concern. One in eight women who have had PID have trouble getting pregnant and/or experience ectopic pregnancies (that's when the embryo implants outside the uterus and isn't viable). This happens because PID can lead to the formation of scar tissue that blocks your reproductive tract, including your fallopian tubes. Many cases of PID are found in women who have no access to reproductive health care or who don't go regularly to the doctor. Basically, when an infection, typically gonorrhea or chlamydia, is either untreated, not treated quickly, or not treated fully, it can spread progressively to all the other parts of your reproductive organs. It can be super unpleasant—long-term. PID symptoms include painful periods, spotting and cramping between periods, pain when having sex or peeing, or just general abdominal pain. It can also produce odd discharge and even fever. The number one way to avoid PID is to practice safer sex. If you're sexually active, you should go for STI screenings regularly, and you should treat any infections you do have quickly and fully.

TEST: PID can be tricky to diagnose. Share your sexual history completely with your doctor. You may need a total pelvic workup. If your doctor needs to take a closer look at your reproductive system, they may even need to perform a laparoscopy—a surgical procedure.

TREATMENT: Fully treat any and all infections you might have. You can be reinfected even if you have been cured from many diseases. Go for regular screenings. If you catch your PID early you can be treated in various ways, but you won't undo the damage that has already been done. Some versions of PID can require surgery.

THREE QUESTIONS

1 I'M SEEING SOMEONE WHO I KNOW IS ALSO SLEEPING WITH OTHER PEOPLE. I AM, TOO. WE ARE ON THE SAME PAGE ABOUT THIS BEING OK. BUT HOW SHOULD WE APPROACH THIS IN TERMS OF SEXUAL SAFETY?

Safer sex in nonmonogamous relationships is possible. One study even showed that people in monogamous partnerships have the same STI risk as those in open relationships. This is mainly due to the fact that around a quarter of people in monogamous relationships aren't actually faithful, coupled with the fact that monogamous couples are less likely to be practicing safer sex. Since you already have an open dialogue about what's up in your relationship, it shouldn't be difficult to extend that to keeping everyone safe. This should involve condoms, properly used, at all times. It may also include taking anal sex off the table as it's riskier than, say, oral sex. If you're both sleeping with just one or two other people, these partners should be in on the safer sex conversations—maybe not all together, but whatever works. Everyone should be getting tested regularly for STIs and sharing this information. If you're sleeping with a lot of other partners, this will increase your risk of contracting an STD. Though it's often trickier, it's still important to share all test results and ask that your partners do the same. Either way, constant use of condoms, testing frequently, and a very open dialogue with your primary partner are essential. Be well.

2 WHY IS ANAL SEX CONSIDERED RISKIER THAN OTHER SEX, OR IS IT?

It is and here's why, according to sexuality educator Francisco Ramirez: the skin in your ass can be more easily torn or experience micro-tears than, say, a self-lubricating vagina. And, by and large, people have less experience around anal sex than other kinds of sex. People don't talk enough about breathing, communication, or testing things out on their own before trying it out with a partner. Combine this with the fact that some people use numbing products—as in lubricants that contain chemicals that numb the ass. If you're numb, you won't know there is pain or that there's something to be aware of. Anal might be riskier for the person receiving rather than the person giving, but this isn't always black-and-white. Let's say the person doing the anal penetrating has something going on on their penis (like an open cut): then they, too, are at risk for contracting a disease. So, if you like anal, test frequently, use condoms, get all lubed up, go slow, communicate, and don't numb yourself. If there is (bad) pain, back off.

3 I'VE BEEN HEARING SOME STIS ARE NOW RESISTANT TO ANTIBIOTICS. WHAT DO I NEED TO KNOW?

Here's the deal: sometimes diseases stop responding to the courses of treatment being used to cure them and the medical community has to find and use something else—or develop an entirely new treatment. In the realm of sexually transmitted diseases, all eyes are on gonorrhea. For a long time, it has been treated with antibiotics. But, at the moment, the bacteria have developed resistance to pretty much every drug used to treat it. Back in the nineties, if you got gonorrhea, your doctor would have prescribed fluoroquinolones (maybe you recognize the drug names ciprofloxacin, ofloxacin, or levofloxacin). But, starting around 2000, fluoroquinolones started being less and less effective in treating the disease in the United States. By 2006, the CDC was no longer recommending fluoroquinolones to treat gonorrhea or associated conditions like pelvic inflammatory disease. So doctors moved on to use cephalosporins, another class of drugs. Today, the medical community worldwide is witnessing the emergence of cephalosporin-resistant gonorrhea. The WHO has data from seventy-seven countries showing that antibiotic resistance is making gonorrhea harder, and sometimes impossible, to treat. Untreated gonorrhea can lead to a whole host of health issues, including an increased chance of getting or giving HIV, infertility, and/or ectopic pregnancies, and it can cause heart and nervous system infections as it spreads to your blood. And gonorrhea is a super common STI. The CDC says 820,000 new infections occur each year in the United States, and less than half are detected and reported to them. Meanwhile, they estimate 246,000 of these infections are resistant to at least one antibiotic.

Doctors and researchers and government agencies all over the world are currently researching new treatment regimens as we've pretty much scraped the bottom of the barrel on remaining antibiotic options that work. The WHO says there isn't a lot that's new and workable in the pipeline. Nothing has yet emerged as a winner. While the researchers do their thing, including working on better monitoring systems and response to drug-resistant strains, here's what you can do: Always use condoms. Get STI testing and have your partners do the same, even if you are witnessing no symptoms. Detection can help prevent the spread of resistant gonorrhea.

CHAPTER 6

THE FINAL ACT:

LET'S TALK ABOUT SEX

So now you know all about the various parts of your vulva and how to take care of it, everything about your period, why masturbation is the bomb, and how not to get pregnant—or an STI. Consider that foreplay. Because the time has come—at long last—to talk about sex. Sex is . . . so fucking good. It has *all* of the feels. It's natural. It's healthy for you—maybe even better than the rest of your wellness routine combined. It's intimate. It makes you glow. It's pleasure.

If you think great sex is all about your vagina, you're mainly wrong. It's physical, but it doesn't happen in a vacuum. Yes, you're rocking about eight thousand nerve fibers while the penis only has four thousand—incredible. But it's not just about your clit, either. Perhaps the most critical organ of female sexuality, according to people who study sex, is the brain. When you're feeling relaxed, good, healthy, strong, confident, aren't stressed, aren't distracted by other worries—silly or not—and you choose to be in the mood for sex, that's when it feels best. Your heart factors in, too. It's useful to be into the person you're in bed with—even for casual hookups. Choosing to clear your

CONSENT

It should go without saying that any sexual encounter should be consensual. As in, you and your partner agree to it, give permission, say yes. "No" can be said at any point during any hookup, without hesitation. So maybe it's *yes, please* to kissing, and grinding, and even oral sex and then *no, thanks* to penetration. Or even no once someone is already inside of you. Or no last week and yes this week and no again next month. You can change your mind and communicate freely, even if it feels awkward or you're worried about hurting someone's feelings. It's truly cool. And both partners should agree on that. Even if both of you have been drinking. Or if someone fell asleep. Or if you feel coerced or otherwise vulnerable. Or if you're with someone you don't know well. Or if you or your partner has had an experience that wasn't consensual in the past. If you're working through the aftermath of sexual assault, emotionally, that's something to discuss, and be mindful of. Only yes means yes. And you have no obligations at any moment—nor does your partner—to do anything you do not want to be doing. Period.

mind and stay present in your body to make way for arousal and sex is not always easy. No mindfulness exercises are. But the rewards are, well, rewarding.

Also, about that word *sex*. It. Does. Not. Have. To. Mean. Penetration. It means whatever you want it to mean. Men who sleep with women may come 95 percent of the time, typically via penis-in-vagina sex, but the majority of women eventually orgasm from nonpenetrative sex. So let's go ahead and redefine sex to mean all the good stuff that gets you off, and not just penetration. Only an estimated 30 percent of women manage to go over the edge exclusively from having a penis inside them. Not in that group? Who cares! Sex does not always look like what happens in movies—Hollywood or porn. People talk, negotiate, take turns, switch positions, bump their heads, laugh, and cry. Not everything happens mutually or at the same time. For women, it's pretty much never the same any time you do it. So figure out what sex means to you, what you want it to mean. It doesn't matter if your middle school sex ed classes only talked about periods and unwanted pregnancy and never about pleasure, or if getting on top of your sexuality hasn't been a focus of yours up until now. That's in the past. You have the power and tools to change that—today. All it takes is a good understanding of how your body works and a partner (or partners) who want to help you play and be played with. And, of course, be safe out there.

DOING IT

Think of everything you have done sexually up until where you are right now, reading these words. Was it desire or intimacy driven? Was it just a series of events where you were trying firsts because you wanted to have done certain things, but with no focus on your own pleasure? Do you know what you want in bed, and are you getting it? Even if you are a fully functioning, orgasmic, ask-for-it-all woman, there's always more to know about your own sexuality. It changes year to year, partner to partner, phase of life to phase of life.

WOMEN VERSUS MEN

For something so fabulous, sex is pretty complicated. Like, if, biologically, the main reason sex exists is procreation, then why oh why don't men and women experience sex the same way? Why are male and female desire generally so different? Does it have something to do with the penis being external/in your face and the vagina being internal/hidden? Are there cultural factors that dictate sexual desire based on gender? And what's the deal with the orgasm gap? American adult women typically have one orgasm for every three their male counterparts manage. Mind-boggling. (Yes, male orgasm is biologically necessary for making a baby and pretty easy to achieve. And, yes, female orgasm is totally unnecessary for getting pregnant and takes a lot more work to achieve—though the possibility of having one might make you more likely to want to have sex.) These are questions that people with lots of degrees have been pondering forever: you know, biologists, doctors, sociologists, psychoanalysts, sex educators, Masters and Johnson, Freud. Research is ongoing. Theories and data abound, but our friend Cindy Gallop, founder of Make Love Not Porn and general all-around badass, cautions against paying too much attention to sex-related data; she feels there isn't enough research for it to be valid. Gallop says this is due to a lack of academic funding for wide-ranging studies coupled with many obstacles to getting unbiased information. Many people don't really like to speak honestly about sex. So even the best researcher has to contend with massive confirmation bias—there's always a difference between what people say they do in bed and what they actually do in bed, and no real way to check those facts.

Still, certain statistics from some studies are too hard to overlook. Like these from a recentish one done by *Cosmopolitan* that concluded straight single women have the fewest orgasms: 57 percent of these women have an orgasm most or every time they have sex with a partner; 95 percent of those women's partners have an orgasm most or every time. Even accounting for some people faking it, or not answering honestly, that's some serious orgasm disparity right there. The same survey has 78 percent of women saying they believe their partners want them to orgasm, but 72 percent say they've had partners climax and not help them finish. You could say a *Cosmo* web poll isn't the height of scientific research but other studies back these figures up, give or take a few percentage points. Here's another data point too interesting to overlook, from another study: when a woman is having sex with a woman, the rate of orgasm goes way up, basically matching that of a straight man having sex with a woman. Guess orgasms don't have to be so hard to come by after all. Women know more about what women want, and when we have sex with men, we may need to say what we want more clearly. Technically and physically we can do it, regardless of whom we prefer to have sex with. What often gets in the way is all the other stuff—desire, situation, emotional state, clued-in partner who prioritizes your pleasure—that's what makes or breaks the female O.

Of course orgasm isn't the end-all be-all of sex. A sexual encounter can be all kinds of hot and enjoyable with no final kaboom. According to some studies, about 10 percent of women are truly incapable of having orgasms. If you feel you're in that realm, we highly suggest masturbation—see chapter three, with or without a vibrator—and, separately, an honest chat with your doctor and maybe even a therapist. All three can help. But there is no denying that orgasms are truly transcendent, so why not make them a goal? As Cindy Gallop puts it, "There's a school of thought that there is too much focus on the orgasm. I think that's all very well but an orgasm is fucking amazing." Amen. Her only caveat here is that if a partner is pressuring you to have an orgasm, that's no good. She thinks all women need to expect a one-to-one orgasm ratio. "Flip the gender," says Gallop. "Imagine if every woman went into every encounter and expected it's her God-given right to come. And imagine if men were like, *It would be really nice but it's OK if it doesn't happen.* Women need to demand one-to-one, even in casual one-night stands. I am very results focused. I speak heteronormatively because I am straight, but this applies to all."

Your own desire—and ultimately your orgasms—will be as unique as you are. But, despite our differences, women can hack good sex a little. Basically it takes desire (wanting to have sex), self-awareness (knowing through masturbation what gets you off), communication (telling a partner what feels good), and letting go (do it!). Great sex can just spontaneously happen, for sure, and when it does, that's a bonus—plus stuff to fantasize about later. But more often than not it's about getting on top of your own sexuality. This takes work, concentration, and finding a partner who is willing to be more focused on your pleasure than his or her own for the time you need. You'll get them back. It's unfair to you and to your partner to passively hand your desire over to them and hope they figure it out. If you have an itch on your back, you have to direct someone to where it needs to be scratched, you know? Taking charge and giving directions will get you your desired results and it will mean your partner isn't frustrated by not knowing how to help you. There are occasional partners with whom the attraction is so electric no words are needed, but most of us need pointers, a road map, or a few tasks to follow. No one likes feeling lost or clueless, and everyone adores positive feedback in the form of your pleasure. There's nothing better than being in bed with someone having a fabulous time with you.

THE PHASES OF SEXUAL BEHAVIOR

A number of years ago, back in the 1960s, the research team Dr. William H. Masters and Virginia E. Johnson (usually just referred to as Masters and Johnson—if you watch the TV show *Masters of Sex*, that's them) came up with these four phases of the sexual response cycle—for both men and women. It's just one model of sexual behavior, but, as of now, it's basically the most well-known one. It's hard to put something so unique into a one-size-fits-all categorization, so this model has plenty of detractors who think it doesn't cover everything it should, including desire, emotional intimacy, and satisfaction. Not everyone is a fan. Thankfully, researchers are still working on adding to this model and coming up with different models that take into account all the myriad differences that make up a woman's sexual experience today. For better or worse, here's the gist of Masters and Johnson's model:

1. **EXCITEMENT:** Desire, you want it, blood is in your various erogenous zones, you're swollen, your heart rate goes up, your skin may flush, your nipples may get hard, maybe your vagina feels wet and more open because increased blood circulation produces fluid. Basically, you're turned on.

2. **PLATEAU:** You're on the edge, every single thing that was happening in phase one gets super intensified. Your clit may even feel too sensitive to touch and actually retracts under its hood to protect itself. Your breathing has likely changed, and is heavier. Your muscles might feel tense. You're wetter, though some women produce more lubrication than others. Some people like to ride this edge for a while in an effort to make the next phase more intense. This can be fun.

3. **ORGASM:** Everything speeds up and intensifies and your muscles are all tense and your skin all flushed and then, usually if your clit has been amply attended to, there's a sweet, sweet release, sometimes super strong, sometimes more mild. Your vagina and even your uterus contract.

4. **RESOLUTION:** Basically back to normal but basking in your afterglow. Some women can rapidly return

from this phase back to the orgasm phase with very little prodding, while men need some time to recover before another round.

ORGASM

It's difficult to define an orgasm. Each one is as different as the women having them. But still we try.

"Think of the absolute best foot massage you've ever had, then multiply that by one hundred."

"It's the ticklish buildup to the biggest sneeze ever, plus the sneeze, and then the best exhaustion postsneeze."

"Toe-curling, heart-pumping, pure and uncontrollable pleasure."

"Blacking out—in the best way possible!"

"Lack of breath, emptiness in the whole body, tingling all over with goose bumps."

"A powerful feeling of amazing sensation, including a falling-over-cliff loss of accumulated erotic tension."

"An involuntary muscle contraction accompanied by whole-body bliss."

"When your body takes over out of your own control, totally adhering to your pleasure, your mind is quiet, and then an explosion."

"Scratching the worst itch ever, it almost hurts it's so itchy, resulting in full-body waves of clenching and releasing—almost spasmic and totally spontaneous."

"Orgasm is the sudden, involuntary release of sexual tension." (This one is from Emily Nagoski, author of *Come As You Are*.)

You can read the overlap in experience here, but also how unique every woman's experience is. Basically, orgasm is a mystery. If you have had one—or a zillion—you know why. It feels different pretty much every time. Some are lovely. Some are thunderstorms. Some change your life. Some are full of emotion. Some are purely physical. Some are sad. Some feel like they come from deep inside. Some can stop your cramps. Some reduce you to tears. Some make you want another one right away because they're not quite enough or because they were so good you want more. And so on. The point is that quality varies; maybe the most consistent thing about them is that each one is its very own thing. Yes, researchers can measure uterine contractions and conclude what is and is not an orgasm, but sorry, all the data-collecting probes in the world can't detect all this wide-ranging nuance. And it's probably easier to have an honest orgasm when there isn't a probe inside of you, anyway. Still, people—amateurs and researchers alike—are busily trying to define the female orgasm.

If you have yet to have an O, and would like to, know that it's within reach. Masturbation helps (see chapter three). As does age—most women get better at it with time and experience. We supposedly peak in our thirties and forties—and then keep going. While the vagina atrophies with menopause, the clitoris does not. So we can be enjoying ourselves for many, many years to come.

Definition-happy people aren't satisfied by just mapping out what an orgasm is. Some like to go a step further and define what kind of orgasm an orgasm is. To us, any orgasm is great—an orgasm is an orgasm, who cares where it's coming from? Too many women wind up feeling like they're not having the "right" kind of orgasm or that their bodies don't work because they read an article that claims they can have twelve different kinds of orgasms and then can't figure out how to make their various "spots" respond a dozen different ways. Which is so wrong on so many levels. Still, if you don't feel like you have to succeed, trying to trigger specific kinds of orgasms can actually be a fun game to play with a partner, especially in long-term relationships once the initial sexual fervor dies down a bit. Can you come from having your breasts touched or kissing alone? Can you have an anal orgasm? Can a fantasy send you over the edge? Can you use yoga breathing techniques to "move" your orgasm from feeling localized in your vulva and push it all over your body? Can you have a blended orgasm—two trigger spots at the same time? Can you even tell? It may be impossible to say when you're in the heat of things. Or, when you're coming you might prefer to just enjoy rather than focus on physiology. Besides, all our parts are pretty interwoven, and many of these spots get touched, prodded, stroked, and jostled throughout the course of a sexual encounter, which is kind of the point. Maybe your exploration won't lead to clearly distinct kinds of orgasms, considering how different any orgasm feels, and how unique our bodies all are, anatomically. But exploration in and of itself can be totally hot. So if you're interested, there's no harm in hunting. See how your body responds—no pressure. With that in mind, here are some of the various kinds of female Os that are supposedly available to have.

Clitoral Versus Vaginal

For a while there, people believed that clitoral orgasms were immature while vaginal ones were mature, (no) thanks to Dr. Sigmund Freud back in, like, 1905. This mainly meant the clit got sadly ignored for far too long and women were made to feel bad about how their bodies functioned if they weren't having so-called vaginal orgasms. Thankfully other researchers eventually came around and said what we clit owners already know: all orgasms are clitoral orgasms, they're not really distinct, and they're awesome. This is an oversimplification of just how heated this debate was and continues to be. If you're interested, there's plenty more stuff to read on the topic. If you're coming from penetration inside your vagina versus direct external clitoral stimulation (oral, rubbing, vibrator, whatever it takes), it's usually because someone or something is hitting some part of your clitoris the right way inside of you—usually the clitoral root. Remember from the diagram on page 18 that the visible clitoral nub is only the tip of the iceberg, and the rest is internal. If your clitoris happens to be close to your vaginal opening, you may have an easier time having orgasms during penetration. Lucky you if you're built that way and/or you've otherwise gotten off from vaginal penetration—statistics show this only happens for about 30 percent of women. Either way, you're going to want some clitoral attention.

G-spot

Named after a German-born gynecologist named Ernst Gräfenberg, who also developed a ring-shaped IUD (busy guy!), this refers to a small spot of erogenous tissue on the front wall of the vagina, basically where it wraps around the urethra. Since it's internal, some people consider a G-spot orgasm a vaginal orgasm. If this is a sensitive spot in your body, you probably already know about it. If it's working, keep at it. But if you feel nothing up around there, it might be of interest to learn that a lot of women agree with you and many doctors believe the G-spot is a myth. One recentish example: in 2012 a urology resident at Yale published an article in the *Journal of Sexual Medicine* saying the G-spot does not exist. He did the research and didn't find the response in women to support it. And yet, other doctors swear it's no myth, and the G-spot is endlessly being studied, with ultrasounds seeking anatomical proof and more, in an attempt to locate it. It kind of boggles the mind

DO YOU SQUIRT?

Squirting, aka female ejaculation, aka gushing, is fluid that gets released from glands adjacent to your pee hole that isn't urine. We know this because scientists have actually studied the chemical composition of the liquid. Squirting can happen during any kind of sexual stimulation (some say it helps to pay a lot of attention to the G-spot, if you feel like you have one), at any point, though some women release the fluid when they orgasm. Squirting has become a thing mainly because of porn, where it's a much-filmed, almost fetishy occurrence. And even though there are a zillion how-to tutorials available on the topic online, plus tons of misinformation, the general medical consensus is either you have the squirting gland or you don't. Even if you're not technically squirting, you may think you are when you experience a lot of wetness. Maybe you had urine in your bladder and it got banged around since it's so close to your clitoris during sex, and you released some. Or maybe you got extra hugely turned on and were at a time in your menstrual cycle where your cervical mucus was copious and that's what made things really wet. Actual squirting fluid, pee, or cervical mucus—it doesn't really matter. If you do gush and that's hot for you and your partner, enjoy!

how much time, energy, and money has been put toward locating this spot, but it's probably because sex is so fun and the idea of such a thing is undeniably intriguing and potentially lucrative. What if? If you do feel something in that area, scientists seeking to explain your response have variously posited that it's the back end of the clitoris, somehow related to anal muscles, or even an internal clitoris. Either way, try sticking your (clean) fingers up there and see what happens—if you sense nothing at twelve o'clock, try three, six, nine, and notice what you feel—or spend some time exploring with your partner. The worst that could happen is that you have a lot of sex while in search of this elusive spot, even if you never find it. Win-win.

A-spot

In the search for spots that set off long-lasting, intense internal orgasms, researchers, specifically a Malaysian doctor named Chua Chee Ann, MD, as recently as 1997, have hit on the anterior fornix. This spot is deeper in the vagina than the G-spot, which has earned it the nickname of the "deep" spot, though there is some debate about where it actually is—some people say it's between the cervix and the bladder, some describe it as being on the same side of the vaginal wall as the G-spot, but higher. Some people say it's on the opposite wall. Others say it's on the curve going toward the cervix. Still others say the "deep" spot isn't the A-spot at all but rather the posterior fornix, whose stimulation can lead to what some call a cervical orgasm. Confused? You're not alone. At least some of this confusion must have to do with the fact that we're all shaped a little differently. But it's also partly why some doctors believe that the A-spot, like the G-spot, is a myth, and what women must actually be feeling is something in their cervix, which is even deeper in the vaginal canal. Maybe it's like a female prostate, maybe not. Maybe it's just where some nerves happen to be bundled, maybe not. Among its varied promises is that touching the A-spot supposedly can lead to "rapid" vaginal lubrication with no foreplay. Sounds promising, but we're never down for eliminating foreplay, and getting way up in there without any lubrication to begin with might be a dicey proposition. As with the G-spot, if you can't find your A-spot, you're not alone. But trying to find it—solo or with someone—could be hot. There's nothing wrong with setting aside time to find what pleasures you with fingers, toys, or a penis; even if you never find what you're supposedly looking for, you'll likely wind up having a blast. Certain positions are more likely than others to reach the A-spot via penetration, like doggie, or missionary, especially if you pull your knees up. And if it turns out you like it deep, like cervical deep, go for it.

HOW TO HAVE AN ORGASM WITH A PARTNER

If we could tell you, we'd be famous! Every single woman is different. The best advice is to know how you have one when you masturbate. Think of pleasure as a discipline. It takes some effort to cultivate. There's no magic formula, but to orgasm with a partner, you have to want it and to let yourself have it. Be in the right mind-set to get aroused and to be open to letting go—including letting go of the expectation that you *have to* have an orgasm. Throwing in the towel if it isn't happening is fine. Here are some general tips and strategies that might get you to where you're trying to go.

- It helps not to be stressed. Try meditating. Or a glass of wine can calm your nerves, but drinking too much will hurt your cause.
- It helps to be into your partner.
- It helps to have a partner who wants to help you orgasm but also isn't pressuring you.
- It helps not to be rushed (though sometimes a quickie is just the thing).

- It helps to tune deeply into what feels amazing and to let it feel amazing, let the focus be on you for the duration.
- It helps to communicate clearly to your partner what's working and what is not working.
- It helps not to mentally go through your to-do list.

And it really, really helps to get as aroused as humanly possible—whatever that takes, including porn, reading erotica, massage, or fantasizing. And, yes, fantasy might mean not thinking about the person in front of you. That does it for some people. If of interest, give it a try. If what gets you really turned on is your own hands or your vibrator, use both. Like oral? Go for it. Try oral with fingers or with a vibrator. Mix it up to surprise your body. Penetration doesn't have to be on the menu if you don't want it. Remember, only some women get off that way. You'll reciprocate—later. Set yourself up for success: Do you like music? Play it. Do you like darkness? Turn off the lights. Block distraction by turning off your phone. A little dry? Use lube. Concerned about smells and tastes? Take a steamy shower together. Try it all. Again and again. It's all pleasure—and it might just work.

U-spot

You may have already noticed when someone was going down on you that the opening to your urethra (that's your pee hole, just above your vaginal opening) can feel pretty good when licked. Some people refer to this as the U-spot. Whatever you want to call it, you can stimulate it either manually or with the tip of a penis with a little lube as well as with a tongue—if it feels good. Just be gentle. It can be pretty sensitive.

MULTIPLES

If you can have more than one orgasm in a row, hats off to you. If you can't and you want to work on "moregasm," go for it. If you don't see the point of more than one, skip to the next section. Technically all women can have multiple orgasms because we don't require what's called a "refractory period" after we come. Men need this to basically regain their strength, while women can keep going and going and going. That said, if you've heard a female friend brag about having one hundred orgasms an hour, that's unrealistic. But who knows. We're all built differently. Go her. In order to be multiply orgasmic you need to be up for taking care of your own pleasure. It's not really the sort of thing your partner alone can make happen for you—though they will likely be psyched to be there as you

DON'T BE FAKE

Apparently 80 percent of women have faked an orgasm in their lifetime. This is a bummer. Faking it means you're not feeling pleasure and you're confusing and miseducating your partner.

So what's standing between you and your own pleasure?

- Are you not into your partner? Find someone else.
- Do you not know what an orgasm feels like? Get to know your own body better through masturbation. Once you've figured out what sends you over the edge, it will be easier to replicate in real time with someone else in the bed. You can teach them your methods. Because, as every sex expert says every time anyone brings up orgasm, most women don't get there from penetration alone. Or you can work your skills while they watch, or otherwise participate—hand them your toy of choice! Whatever works.
- Is it medical? Are you too stressed or depressed to bother with orgasm? Are you on a medication that is making it harder to reach orgasm? Talk to your doctor. And talk to your partner! Honesty is the best policy.

And remember: this is about you. Orgasm is not so you can make a partner happy, though it's of course fun to share—especially with a partner who wants to help you get there. It's because it feels good and is healthy—for you. So don't fake it.

try. If it's not just happening to you naturally, enticing your body to have multiples usually requires some self-exploration via masturbation before taking your party trick public.

The two basic kinds of multiple orgasms are sequential and serial. Sequential means you have one orgasm right after the other, with rest time in between. You go through all those phases of arousal Masters and Johnson described, then do it again. Serial means you have them one after the other, back-to-back, without ever fully recovering from the tail end of your first O. You sort of ride the end of the wave of one, while you're still aroused, and there is still blood engorging all the right places. You apply the pressure it will take to whatever spot or spots gets you off the easiest—hi, clitoris—to try to bring about a second or third or however many more orgasms. Some studies have shown that multiples are more likely to happen if you're stimulating more than one erogenous spot at once. If you do have a sensitive G-spot, that's a good place to try to trigger a multiple. If you've had a really whopping first orgasm, more may not be of interest. Or sometimes your clitoris will feel too sensitive to continue touching. Try it a bunch of different ways to see what works for you, if you're curious. You never know what you might come up with.

THE PEOPLE YOU MEET

Partnered sex is all about partners. When you're on your own, you know how to do you. When other people enter the scene, the realm of possibility blossoms. Every partner brings something different to the bedroom. Whether you're into casual hookups, trying a threesome for the first time, are in the happy bliss of a new fling, or have been with someone for years, your sex life will vary—obviously. And communication—open, honest, and constant—is always the key to satisfaction.

WHO DO YOU LIKE?

Sexual orientation is no longer an either/or scenario. If you feel you're 100 percent homosexual or heterosexual, OK, good to know who you are and what you like. But research shows that a strictly binary sex model is a thing of the past. Sexuality is just more fluid than that. For a while, scientists were defining sexual orientation based on a scale from zero to six that was created by sexologist Alfred Kinsey back in the 1940s. So if you had sex primarily with people of your own gender, you'd be like a five or a six on that scale. But if you were mainly having sex with the opposite gender, you'd be in the zero-to-one range. At some point it became obvious that this wasn't a particularly modern approach. If you're someone who still wants to know where you fall on a scale (versus just enjoying yourself), check out the Klein Sexual Orientation Grid, created in the late 1970s, which takes into account the fluidity of sexuality, emotional and social preferences, and even considers how sexuality changes over time. Then there's an even newer scale, called the Purple-Red scale of attraction. A scientist didn't create it, but it's pretty interesting. It denotes attraction type (from aromantic to hypersexual) plus orientation (homo to hetero).

Sex is an exploration, an experiment. So explore any which way that will arouse you—as long as you're being safe. Bisexual, pansexual, asexual, questioning, it's all good. Also, say you consider yourself a heterosexual woman but you love to masturbate to lesbian erotica or you get super excited watching two men have sex. That doesn't "mean" anything, other than that's what gets you off. Fantasy is fantasy. And if you choose at some point to act on your fantasy, that's up to you.

COMMUNICATION

We know we've been going on and on about how masturbation is the key to having awesome partnered sex. Hopefully you've internalized this by now. But communication is just as, if not more, critical—and the two combined are unstoppable. You need to be able to tell anyone you're getting down with what you want and how. If you can't speak up, the other person is left in the dark just guessing. And that's no way to get on top of your pleasure. In general, women take a minute to get turned on. It's not that men don't need foreplay, and don't need to express how best to turn them on. They do. But in the give and take that happens in any sexual encounter, they usually need a little less help. And part of what can get them going is watching you enjoy yourself. So it's all interrelated. You and your partner will have to decide when it's easier to talk about sex—before, during, after, outside of the bedroom, in the shower, while cooking dinner or drinking tequila. Whatever. But do talk about it. Talk about what turns you on. Share your masturbation techniques. Talk about what you want to do to each other. Talk about what you have done to each other that felt good, that worked well. Relive the fun. Tell each other how you like to pace things. Express the difference between when you're just enjoying yourself versus when you want to start building to an orgasm. Ask questions. Listen. Set boundaries. Don't overthink it, just do it. No one is a mind reader. You don't have to start with anything too graphic or specific if you don't want to. It can be directional—left, right, up, down. But ultimately the more you share, the better it can be.

KEEPING IT CASUAL

Enjoying sex with someone you don't know is kind of like an art form. For a number of reasons, data shows, random hookups don't usually result in orgasms for women. Studies on this sort of thing are limited, but basically women tend to prioritize men's pleasure and men tend to be more interested in themselves when they don't know their partner and aren't emotionally involved with them. Still, getting off casually is possible. Say you just met on Raya or at a bar or a friend's wedding, and you feel a spark and want to go for it. Just do what you'd do with any partner: be safe, communicate, and don't be afraid to touch yourself as they touch you. If you almost come but don't, so what? Every encounter you have—life changing or not—helps you know you better. And it enhances the next one. And, if the person is worth pursuing beyond a one-night stand, there's always next time. If at first you don't succeed . . .

That said, if you're getting down with a casual hookup and it's not going well, stop at any point. Anecdotally, lots of people—men and women—"finish off" what they started with strangers because they're already doing it. There's no reason or obligation to finish anything you're not into.

RELATIONSHIPS

The research is clear: women in relationships have more orgasms than women not in relationships. In male/female relationships, the orgasm gap shrinks. Female orgasms are by and large what are referred to as "context dependent." And men, statistically, make better partners when they care about and know their girlfriend (or wife). It's also clear that when two people have been together for a while, things can slow down. But there are endless ways to bring back the fire. Sexuality is, after all, lifelong. So while the days of literally feeling electricity on your skin when your partner touches you might be in the past, the spark is always there. Deciding with your partner to make sex a top concern—something you care about and want to work on together—and having open communication will help you tap into it as the months and even years roll by.

Being honest with your partner when your new relationship energy fades and things slow down, sharing that disappointment together, and continuously finding playful ways to be sexual are all important parts of maintaining long-term relationships. Maybe you never felt comfortable bringing a toy into the bedroom during your first years together, or watching porn, or trying a new position, or looking for any of the various supposed orgasm trigger spots—G, A, U, or whatever some sex researcher comes up with next—these are all great ways to tap back into your initial spark. It's up to you both to add to it and keep it going. There may have been a time when the idea of "scheduling" sex to make sure you had it at least weekly would have been beyond comprehension. But then maybe you or your partner got a new job, or went back to grad school, or you're hooking up with someone who has a kid, and then suddenly it all makes sense. Sexuality can fade, and all kinds of life-shifting busy-making experiences can get in its way—illness, family issues, work. If you and your partner can choose to make your shared sexuality a mutual priority, to stress its importance, then it will always be there for you, even if it has been dormant for a while.

Sex is just as good for you at any age, any stage of life, any phase of the game. Try out a fantasy or commit to trying something new. This does not have to mean a threesome if that's not your thing. It can be as simple (and awesome) as doing a new breathing technique. Dr. Jill Blakeway, founder of the YinOva Center in New York City and author of *Sex Again: Recharging Your Libido*, suggests something called looping. Basically you use a four-count yoga or meditational breath (four-count inhale, four-count exhale) to try to unlocalize your orgasms out of your vagina, thread the energy around, and create a whole-body orgasm. "Orgasm has become very local," she says. "And a lot of women don't orgasm at all. It's about stagnation and not being able to let go. Even when they do, it's often quite local. It's possible to spread that feeling throughout your body, looping energy up your spine and down the front." An advanced version of the looping involves syncing your breath up with your partner. Give it a whirl. Even if you don't manage a full-body orgasm, chances are you will be present, not distracted, in the moment, and you and your partner will have a good laugh together. That's a lot better than going through your to-do list or wondering who will do the dishes while your partner is going down on you. If looping isn't your thing, find something that is. Slow things down. Try tantra. Spend time touching every part of your vulva—with no other expectations—to see what's sensitive. Work toward multiple orgasms, or extending your orgasms. The amounts of games to play are really endless. It just depends on how playful you want to be on any given day. Keeping sex alive in a long-term relationship is a choice and a learned skill. It's well worth the effort.

ADD-ONS

Sex is natural. All you need is your own naked body. But sometimes a little gear can enhance the proceedings. Here are a few ways to take things up a notch.

LUBE

Lube is the best thing ever. Some women self-lubricate copiously, some do not. And some do some of the time, but not all of the time. For whenever you're not producing as much as you'd like, there is personal lubricant available for purchase. And purchase you should. But first! There are a number of things to consider. You cannot use any oil-based lubrication with a condom; they will break down the latex. They will also break down the plastic on some sex toys. So even if you're an I-use-coconut-oil-for-everything kind of person, the buck stops here if you're also using condoms and toys. "Water-based is like O negative; it works with everything. A lot of people consider it to be healthiest," says Alexandra Fine, cofounder and CEO of Dame Products. She always suggests water-based lube for use with her vibrators.

Then you want to know what's in the lubricant, besides being water-based. Is it vagina-friendly? Anything that would irritate or otherwise harm your vagina is not friendly. Read ingredient lists and ask questions to know what's going inside your body.

Avoid These Ingredients

- **Propylene glycol**

This petrochemical is used as a humectant in lube, which means it can draw and seal in moisture. It's also found in automatic and hydraulic brake fluid. It's used for industrial antifreeze and deicing solution for cars, airplanes, and boats and as a solvent by the paint and plastic industries. It's known that it may be harmful by ingestion, by inhalation, or through skin contact and that it's irritating to the eyes and skin. It can damage vaginal and rectal tissue.

- **Paraben preservatives**

Parabens are currently under medical scrutiny as they have been identified as estrogenic and disruptive of normal hormone functions; studies are linking them with breast cancer tumors.

- **Polyethylene glycol (PEG)**

Used as a thickener in lubes, it strips the skin's natural moisture. An eye irritant and possible carcinogen, PEG can produce severe acidosis, central nervous system damage, and congestion.

- **Glycerin**

This viscous liquid is a by-product of soap manufacturing. There is such a thing as natural glycerin, extracted from vegetables, but the more commonly used version is manufactured synthetically. It, and other petrochemical ingredients found in lubricants (plus vaginal washes and douches), can damage the cellular tissue that protects your body from bacterial vaginosis (see page 37), a common infection that can be treated with antibiotics but typically reoccurs. Petrochemical ingredients, including glycerin, disrupt the normal balance of bacteria in the vagina, making way for harmful bacteria to take over. This results in itching, burning, a foul smell, and gray discharge. Two in five women have BV, but most don't even know they have it. A BV infection can make women 60 percent more susceptible to HIV and other STIs, and puts them at an increased risk for pelvic inflammatory disease (PID, see page 182).

What to Look For

- Third-party certified organic ingredients, including aloe vera
- Safe thickeners
- Safer preservatives
- Ideally you want a lube that's similar in pH to your vagina so it won't set off any sort of imbalance or infections with the above harsh chemicals or fragrance (see page 27).

Then you of course want to know how a lube performs—is it sticky, how does it feel on your skin, what kind of glide does it give you, and how long does it last? Does it work well for anal, if you like anal? Also: does it smell and can you safely eat it, if that's your thing? Is it easy to wipe up and off your body? Once you have a lube you like, use it copiously. There's no need to be stingy or to trot it out only for special occasions. Sex should not hurt. If it does, there are a number of possible reasons why. Many can be fixed by lubrication. It can increase pleasure, minimize condom breakage, and even reduce the risk of STIs. If any lubricant is irritating you, discontinue use pronto. Women who have pain with penetration that lubrication does not help shouldn't feel alone. There are options. Both gynecologists and physical therapists who specialize in pelvic pain syndromes can help.

TOYS

Adding a vibrator to partnered sex can be a great idea, especially if that's what helps you enjoy yourself. Again, communicate. Tell your partner you're bringing a toy into the mix and make sure they're into that. Or ask your partner about how a toy would, well, rub them, and let them know it would make you feel jazzed. There is no one right way to tell a partner you want to introduce a toy. "It's a dance between two unique individuals," says Dame Products' Alexandra Fine. "These are conversations to have outside of the bedroom when you're less vulnerable."

Then it's a matter of what toy to use. You could just bring your favorite vibrator into the bedroom (see page 90). Or you can look into partner toys—there's no one-size-fits-all. There are toys where one partner is wearing it and the other partner has a remote control or can work it via a phone app. There are others that women can wear during penetrative sex for hands-free clitoral stimulation, which is hard to get (shout out to Dame Products' Eva!). You can obviously use your hand, but when you're moving up and down and someone else is moving in and out, it can be a little difficult. "They are sprinkles on top," says Fine. Toys don't take over the experience but enhance it.

PROPS

For couples who are interested in trying different positions, positioners can be useful. If you're up for a little role-playing, there is no end to the costumes and tools available. Spend some time with your partner in a store—in person or online—and see what turns you on. Whips, chains, clamps, feathers, handcuffs, blindfolds, restraints, outfits—from classic costumes to fuzzy unicorn onesies. Do whatever gets you getting after it.

MIXING IT UP

Some people prefer all their sex on what's considered the "kinky" side. Or some couples dip their toes into what's new and different to them to change things up. Switching things up can be as easy as changing venues, times of day, or positions—it doesn't have to mean you're suddenly swinging or going to dungeons, unless you want to. It can be anything from adding anal or (more) oral to the mix or acting out a fantasy. As with all fun sex, communication is key. Share a desire you've never acted on. Help your partner do something he or she has been yearning to try. Dream up what you want to do together, then do it.

BACK TO NATURE

Getting outside—with or without the possibility of getting caught—can be a blast. But even just getting out of bed and onto the floor, your kitchen counter, or your couch can help bust you out of a rut. Being playful is key, but try not to get caught; you could actually face a fine. Come prepared (blankets, condoms, wipes—no one wants sand in their vagina), and try these spots:

- In the woods, on a hike
- On the beach, day or night under the stars

- Water works: a shower, bath, pool, or hot tub, or rainstorm
- Urban rooftops

POSITIONS

There are so many different ways to have sex. We all tend to do the positions we know bring us to fruition. Makes sense. Even if you're actively trying new ones, you may still want to finish off in your favorite position for the best possible outcome. But don't get lazy. Try something different from time to time; it might just bring on some new feels. Keep in mind that many of the positions you see in porn or in the *Kama Sutra* aren't really comfortable, but they can be hot. At the very least they're good for a laugh and are amusing to try. And consider changing up what you do even in your favorite positions. Do you like to be on top? Get on top for oral, too. Are you usually in the dark or in candlelight? Try lights on. Are your eyes usually closed? Open wide.

ANAL

If ass play isn't on your regular list of stuff you do, and you're interested in giving it a go, you'll need two things. First up is condoms. The skin up your ass is incredibly fragile, even more so than the tissue in the vagina. It can tear easily, which puts you at higher risk for contracting STIs, including HIV. And second is lubrication. The ass does not produce its own lube, unlike vaginas. Use lube copiously. You can start with fingers or toys or you can go straight to a penis; either way, go slow. Like really, really slow. Relaxation, breathing, and communication are critical. So is hygiene—hands and toys need to be washed when you're done playing—especially if you're moving on to any kind of vaginal play. If you're not quite sure what you're doing, read up on anal before you try. If you love it, keep going. But if you don't, no worries. If your partner loves anal and you don't, or vice versa, that's a conversation you'll need to have.

PORN

Women make up around 26 percent of the visitors of Pornhub .com. And we have our own way of watching: 80 percent of women watch on smartphones or tablets, and are 34 percent less likely than men to use a desktop computer to view. If you and your partner like to watch porn together, enjoy it. Talk openly about what turns you on, what you find attractive, what you want to see that will arouse you. Seeing other people go at it or role-play a fantasy can really add to all aspects of partnered sex—from getting hot to completion.

Keep in mind that, as discussed on page 100, porn is like wrestling: It's staged. It's unrealistic entertainment created solely as entertainment. "It objectifies sex," says Dr. Laurie Betito, a clinical psychologist and sex therapist. "It reduces it to basic genitals. It's missing all the other elements of good sex, like intimacy." And yet, watching it can really warm some people up. Dr. Laurie runs a sexual wellness portal for Pornhub.com and she says it's fine to compartmentalize when enjoying porn. Fantasy is just fantasy, it's OK to be turned on by whatever turns you on. And, no, not all porn is violent against women, though many people, women included, have fantasies about women being controlled. Still others prefer women dominate. "Don't read so much into it," says Dr. Laurie. Or stage and film your own video with your partner.

Visuals not your thing? Give erotica a try—take turns reading out loud to each other. If you hate porn, or dislike any part of what you think it stands for, ignore it. It's not for you. If your partner loves it and you don't, then it probably won't be something you do together frequently. It can be a private thing, as long as it doesn't take away from the couple. Talk it through with your partner.

ROLE-PLAYING

The point of a couple role-playing is to act out within the confines of your relationship. Part of the fun here is getting your partner to tell you what he or she wants, and then being open to helping them experience this with you. You might be surprised at what you learn about someone you thought you knew in and out—plus what you wind up doing. The flip side of this is letting go enough to vocalize what you want, and trusting your partner to let you have this experience in real life. The actual acting out can be as true to your fantasy as you want it to be, or it can be a lesser version of things. Let's say your partner has been harboring a desire to be dominated. You could literally go out and buy an entire rubber-clad wardrobe, or you could just do a little light bondage, and play a little with whips and eventually go deeper in if you both like it. Whatever works for both of you. In this realm, communication is the high priestess. Don't be shy.

OPEN RELATIONSHIPS

Maybe your ultimate fantasy is to be with partners outside your couple. Or to be with your partner and other partners at the same time. Or you'd love to have sex with another woman—with or without your partner present. All valid desires. Depending on the nature of your primary relationship, this can all be in reach. Many people have open relationships or understandings with their partners about sex outside of the relationship. It's really up to the two of you to decide what's OK with both of you. Communication has to be free-flowing and there should be no coercion going on from either partner. This is a mutual decision that should not be made lightly. But it can for sure work if you're both all in.

THREE QUESTIONS

1 HOW COME I AM WET WHEN I AM NOT EVEN REMOTELY TURNED ON?

When your genital response and your arousal differ, that's called arousal nonconcordance. And it can feel totally random. It happens because genital response is actually linked to sex-related stuff, while arousal happens in the brain. Like, someone touches your breasts, so your genitals respond by self-lubricating. But it does not mean you're enjoying having your breasts touched or are aroused. Arousal nonconcordance can also happen the other way, too—you can feel very aroused and be totally dry. Sexual arousal isn't about what your genitals are doing, as confusing as that sounds. It's hard to wrap your mind around. If a man is turned on, there's usually an erection. So we all assume wetness in women is similar; it means you're good to go. Actually, according to Emily Nagoski, sex educator and author, there is a 50 percent overlap between how erect a guy's penis is and how turned on he feels. But for women, she says, there is a mere 10 percent overlap between what her genitals are doing and how aroused she feels. So, ignore your wetness or your dryness—and let your partner know to ignore it, too. You know when you're aroused or not aroused, be sure to communicate that with your partner. And for when you're dry but very interested, there's lube.

2 I LOVE ORAL, BUT I HATE GIVING BLOW JOBS. IS IT OK TO TAKE AND NOT GIVE?

Such a good question. Flip it around—how would you feel if your partner wanted to take and not give? Ultimately it's something you need to talk to your partner about—openly and honestly. There are times you may feel up to doing what you don't love because it makes a partner happy. Or it may be a total embargo, and you need to work through that with the very person who won't be getting any blow jobs. With any luck, you've found a person who can personally take it or leave it and loves to go down on women—they're out there. Or you've found someone who wants to understand what you don't like and how to make the experience more tolerable for you. Is he taking too long? Would you prefer a little manscaping? Are you gagging? You could also work together to set limits—a few a month or just a little bit as foreplay but not to fruition. What we do for our partners is a bit of a dance. Open conversation is critical.

3 I'M SO INTO MY BOYFRIEND. HE'S GREAT IN EVERY WAY—WE GET ALONG, WE LIKE THE SAME THINGS. IT'S KILLING ME THAT THE SEX IS NOT SO GREAT. IS THERE ANYTHING I CAN DO?

Yes, of course, there are things you can do! There is some expectation if sparks are flying all over the place then everything in the bedroom will follow suit, but this just isn't always the case. Maybe you're both inexperienced, or maybe he is. Or maybe neither of you have been with partners who were really up front about expressing needs and saying what feels good. So now that you have such a great guy, speak up about what you want him to do to and with you, and ask him what he enjoys and wants from you. That's a good way to frame the conversation, because certainly no one wants to hear they're not doing it for their girlfriend. It can be a tricky topic to bring up for sure, so maybe try chatting when you're not naked and in the middle of things, and don't forget to tell him a few things he does that you do really like. Chances are he will be relieved you're broaching the subject. You may even take it a step further and share fantasies you'd like to try together. If it turns out you're truly not sexually compatible, at least you will both have tried your best to make it work.

JOIN THE VAGINA REVOLUTION

OK, OK, enough reading. Now it's time for action. So go on, get on top of your sexual and reproductive health. Continue to educate yourself about your body and how it works. Get cliterate. Treat yourself well. Go to the doctor regularly. Ask questions. Think through your birth control options. Talk openly and honestly with your partners—and even your friends and family—about sex. A lot. Invest in a new vibrator. Embrace the glory that is (organic) lube. Read labels on any products that come on, into, or near your vagina—from period products to bodywash. See if you can find your G-spot (or not). Work on being "moregasmic," because #lifegoals. Be smart. Be safe. Carry condoms wherever you roam. And, above all, enjoy yourself—as much and as often as you want.

RESOURCES

Bookmark-worthy

Power to Decide, the campaign to prevent unplanned pregnancy, Bedsider.org

Planned Parenthood, PlannedParenthood.org

The Guttmacher Institute, Guttmacher.org

The Kinsey Institute, KinseyInstitute.org

Centers for Disease Control and Prevention, cdc.gov

Ask Dr. Angela, AskDrAngela.com

Make Love Not Porn, MakeLoveNotPorn.tv

OMGYES, OmgYes.com

Our Library

S.E.X: The All-You-Need-to-Know Sexuality Guide to Get You Through Your Teens and Twenties by Heather Corinna

What's Up Down There by Lissa Rankin

Come As You Are: The Surprising New Science That Will Transform Your Sex Life by Emily Nagoski

Pussy: A Reclamation by Regena Thomashauer

Girls & Sex: Navigating the Complicated New Landscape by Peggy Orenstein

Sex Again: Recharging Your Libido by Jill Blakeway

Woman: An Intimate Geography by Natalie Angier

ACKNOWLEDGMENTS

I would like to thank the thousands of women who have opened themselves up to me about their sexuality, periods, relationships, and pleasure over the last four years. This book would not have been possible without them. Similarly, I'd like to thank all the women who have come before me and fought for women's reproductive rights and equality. Women like Gloria Steinem and Cecile Richards are a few examples of the many who have made it possible for me to do the work that I do and for a book like this to be welcomed into the world. Additionally, my work at Sustain and on this book would never have happened if my parents hadn't constantly encouraged me to push boundaries, challenge the system, and approach everything I do in life with honesty and courage. Thank you, Jeffrey and Sheila, for enabling me to do the work I believe in, and to fight for what I think is right, even if it means explaining to eighty-year-old relatives that your daughter does in fact sell condoms. I'd also like to thank my partner, Stephen Oshman, for supporting me endlessly in the work that I do, and for being the rock that grounds me but also teaches me balance. Having a partner who not only accepts you for who you are but pushes you to be better, work harder, and pursue your passion is something I am lucky to have, so thank you, Stephen (aka Osh). Last, but certainly not least, I'd like to thank Alexandra Zissu for the many years of bringing my ideas to life through the written word, for making me laugh and gasp on a daily basis, and for being an incredible example of how to raise two feminists in a challenging world.

—Meika Hollender

I would like to thank my lucky stars for having two little (planned!) girls I can share all this critical information with. I send long-term relationship love to their hypersupportive and game-for-anything father, Olli Chanoff. I'm also indebted to both the administration of my high school, which somehow let me set up a condom program way back in the day, and to my sex-positive, fantastically un-prudish parents. But the deep spot of gratitude is reserved for Meika Hollender—her strength, poise, conviction, persistence, and humor make her a joy to collaborate with on any project.

—*Alexandra Zissu*

Meika and Alexandra would both like to thank Michele Martin, Sharon Bowers, and Diana Ventimiglia for helping make this book a reality.

We'd also like to thank, in no particular order:

Dr. Angela Jones
Dr. Nathalie Feldman
Dr. Lauren MacAfee
Ginny Ehrlich
Francisco Ramirez, MPH
Carrie Mumah
Dr. Laurie Betito
Dr. Jill Blakeway, DACM, LAc
Alexandra Fine
Cindy Gallop
Chrystie Heimert
Kate Fraser
Samantha Bloom
Cindy Ratzlaff
Karen Adelson

John Paul Jones
John Vairo
Lisa Litwack
Jaime Putorti
Melissa Rodgers
Jean Anne Rose
Liz Psaltis
Erica Ferguson
Vera Papisova
Kat Oshman
Alexandra Scranton
Cara Bedick
Lara Blackman
Susan Moldow
Tara Parsons
David Falk
Meredith Vilarello
Kelsey Manning
Abigail Novak

ABOUT THE AUTHORS

Meika Hollender is the cofounder of Sustain Natural, a new brand of sexual and reproductive wellness products for women. She is also the creator of #GetOnTop, a national campaign aimed at getting women to take control of their sexual health. She received her MBA from New York University's Stern School of Business, where she was the president of the Social Enterprise Association. Meika has also done stints at the brand strategy and design firm Sterling Brands and at Johnson & Johnson as a sustainability associate. She writes frequently on sexual health issues and advocacy for publications including *Refinery29* and is the coauthor of the book *Naturally Clean*. Through Sustain's 10%4Women initiative, she is proud to work closely with Planned Parenthood. Meika was also recently named one of Fast Company's Most Creative People in 2017, and was listed on *Forbes'* 30 Under 30 list.

Alexandra Zissu is a writer and an editorial consultant. She's the author of *The Conscious Kitchen* and coauthor of *Planet Home*, *The Complete Organic Pregnancy*, and *The Butcher's Guide to Well-Raised Meat*. Her stories have appeared in *The New York Times*, *New York Magazine*, *The New York Observer*, *Women's Wear Daily*, *Teen Vogue*, *Details*, and *Bon Appétit*, among many other publications.